PRIVILEGE *and* POLICY

A HISTORY OF COMMUNITY CLINICS IN SASKATCHEWAN

PRIVILEGE *and* POLICY

A HISTORY OF COMMUNITY CLINICS IN SASKATCHEWAN

by Stan RANDS

REVISED EDITION

Edited by

Gregory P. MARCHILDON

& Catherine LEVITEN-REID

University of Regina

CPRC PRESS

Library and Archives Canada Cataloguing in Publication
Rands, Stan, 1909–1985
Privilege and policy : a history of community clinics in Saskatchewan / Stan Rands.

(Canadian Plains reprint series, 1208-9680 ; 15)
Includes index.
Also issued in electronic format.
ISBN 978-0-88977-290-8

1. Clinics—Saskatchewan—History. 2. Community health services—Saskatchewan—History. 3. Medical care—Saskatchewan—History. 4. Doctors' Strike, Sask., 1962. I. University of Regina. Canadian Plains Research Center II. Title. III. Series: Canadian Plains reprint series ; 15

RA983.A4S27 2012 362.12'097124 C2012-901775-2

Library and Archives Canada Cataloguing in Publication
Rands, Stan, 1909-1985
Privilege and policy [electronic resource] : a history of community clinics in Saskatchewan / Stan Rands.

(Canadian Plains reprint series, 1208-9680 ; 15)
Includes index.
Electronic monograph issued in EPUB format.
Also issued in print format.
ISBN 978-0-88977-291-5

1. Clinics—Saskatchewan—History. 2. Community health services—Saskatchewan—History. 3. Medical care—Saskatchewan—History. 4. Doctors' Strike, Sask., 1962. I. University of Regina. Canadian Plains Research Center II. Title. III. Series: Canadian Plains reprint series (Online) ; 15

RA983.A4S27 2012 362.12'097124 C2012-901776-0

Contents

Index prepared by Adrian Mather, AMindexing, Edmonton, AB.

We acknowledge the financial support of the Government of Canada through the Canada Book Fund for our publishing activities.

We acknowledge the Government of Saskatchewan, through the Grants to Publishers Fund, for its financial support.

Printed in Canada.

Introduction to the 2012 Edition: Community Clinics and Stan Rands's Struggle for the Transformation of Health Care in Canada

Gregory P. Marchildon

Stan Rands and the Doctors' Strike of 1962

The doctors' strike in July 1962 marked the difficult birth of universal medical care (medicare) in Saskatchewan. However, it was the Saskatoon Agreement, the subsequent deal between the provincial government and organized medicine which ended the strike, that would ultimately set the template for universal medicare throughout Canada. As explained years later by Allan Blakeney, one of the key ministers in the Co-operative Commonwealth Federation (CCF) government responsible for introducing medicare, the essence of the Saskatoon Agreement involved a major concession on both sides: organized medicine agreed to stop fighting the establishment of universal medical care insurance, and in return the provincial government agreed not "to try to change in a radical way the manner in which medical care was delivered by physicians."[1] While a single source of public payment replaced individual private payments, doctors would continue to deliver medical services in the same way through their private practices.[2] This middle point between an internally coordinated public health system and a private health insurance system would eventually become known as a single-payer system.[3]

It was precisely this compromise that so vexed Stan Rands in the wake of the 23-day doctors' strike. A committed socialist and communitarian, Rands wanted universal medicare to be a policy that would transform the delivery of health care, not merely change the funding mechanism, as important as this was to ensuring that access would be based on medical need rather than ability to pay. He wanted a particular type of co-operative group practice—the community clinic—to supplant private physicians as the dominant mode of delivering primary care. He wanted the consumer of health services to control these new clinics and redress the traditional inequality of the doctor-patient relationship. And he wanted salary to replace the fee-for-service method of payment so that physicians would quit treating health care as a commodity and instead ensure that patients received adequate preventative care as well as curative services. In other words, he wanted medicare to transform the very nature of primary care, and the CCF government's focus on changing the payment system did not, in his view, go nearly far enough.[4]

Rands never fully accepted the argument, posed by Tommy Douglas, the CCF premier of Saskatchewan from 1944 until 1961, that medicare had to be introduced in two distinct phases, the first removing "the financial barrier between those giving the

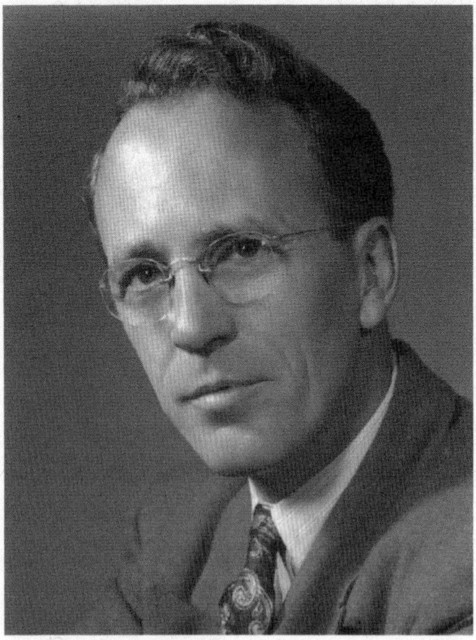

T.C. ("Tommy") Douglas, Premier of Saskatchewan, 1944–61 (SAB R-WS15159-1).

service and those receiving it," and the second "to reorganize and revamp the whole delivery system."[5] From Douglas's perspective, fiscal and political reality necessitated moving in stages. His government took 15 years after it implemented universal hospital insurance to introduce universal medical care insurance. Douglas always wanted the majority of doctors to buy into the changes, and felt that once they had become accustomed to the new funding system, they would eventually be convinced to practice medicine differently. Although he would not bend on the principle that payments for medical services be financed out of government revenues rather than individual payment, Douglas was willing to compromise on the question of whether family doctors should work on salary in group practices or receive a fee for each service in traditional sole physician practices in the expectation that physicians would voluntarily change the way they practised.[6]

Rands disagreed with the premise of this compromise. He felt that the business community and the majority of physicians would permanently oppose both sets of reform and that implementing funding reforms without major changes in delivery and physician payment would only give organized medicine the tools to eventually undercut the funding reform and obstruct the community clinics and their alternative model of primary health care. However, if the government was not prepared to lead the way in this transformation as it was introducing the first phase of medicare, Rands felt that the minimum it could do was at least support the community clinic movement so it could provide an alternative model of delivery to the residents of Saskatchewan, and act as a beacon for future health reforms. Instead, in his view, the provincial government, in the weeks and months following the Saskatoon Agreement, did not go far enough to help the clinics recruit new doctors from the United Kingdom —most local doctors being unwilling to break with the leaders of their own political organization. Worse was the government's extreme reticence to provide alternate forms of remuneration, especially salary, to clinic doctors.

The conventional way to see the medicare battle of the early 1960s is as a titanic struggle between the CCF government and organized medicine, but the reality was more complicated. In particular, there were very deep divisions in both pro- and anti-medicare camps. For example, while the vast majority of doctors appeared to support the hard-line position of their own leadership, the reality was that family doctors in rural Saskatchewan were far less certain of the rightness of their cause, and far less willing to quit serving individuals who were also their neighbours and friends than the urban specialists who dominated their political organization.[7]

Compared to the anti-medicare camp, the split in the pro-medicare camp went much deeper which Rands exposes in considerable depth. The CCF government, in particular cabinet and its most senior advisors in the bureaucracy, found itself at loggerheads with a small but determined group of socialists who, while willing to support the CCF on some common policy objectives, were ultimately skeptical about the CCF's real, as opposed to rhetorical, commitment to fundamental social change. Indeed, many socialists believed that the CCF's desperate efforts to appeal to voters along with its first experience with power in Canada—Tommy Douglas's government in Saskatchewan—had merely served to water down the CCF's original ambitions.[8]

The transformative agenda of democratic leftists such as Rands focused on three main goals, all of which were most prominent in the original CCF manifesto of 1933 but some were muted in subsequent electoral platforms in the 1940s and 1950s. The first was eventually replacing private ownership with either public or co-operative ownership: in other words, getting rid of the profit motive in human affairs. The second was changing the form and content of education so that it would be potentially accessible to all members of society at any stage of life: this learning could then be used by ordinary citizens to criticize and overturn institutionalized inequalities. The third goal was transforming health care from a market commodity to a right so that there would be no financial barriers to care and the relationship between provider and patient would be based solely on health considerations. At various times in his life, Rands was focused on one or the other of these goals, but in the decade following the doctors' strike, he worked on all three simultaneously.

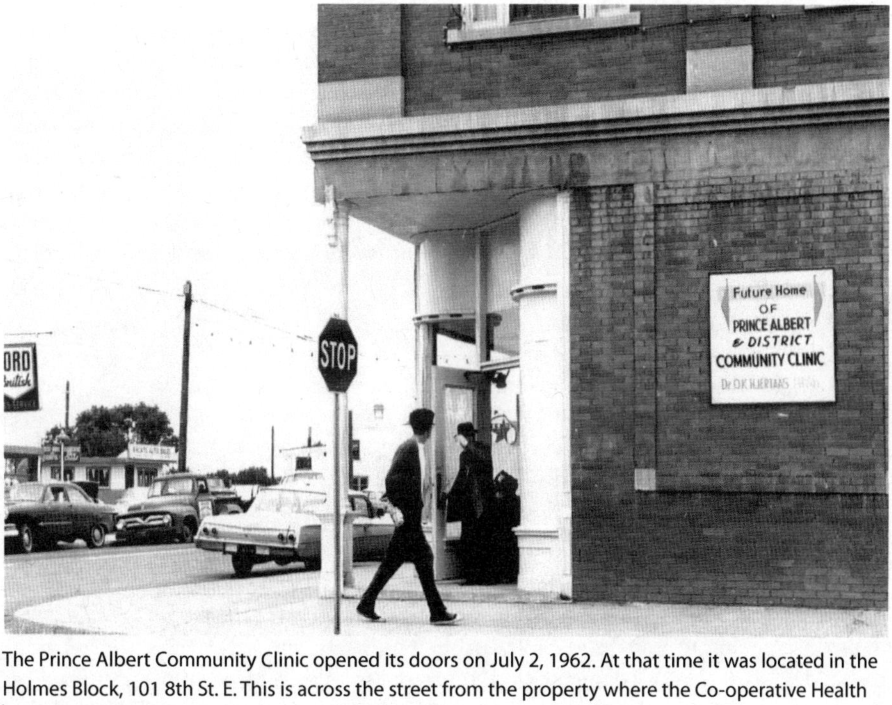

The Prince Albert Community Clinic opened its doors on July 2, 1962. At that time it was located in the Holmes Block, 101 8th St. E. This is across the street from the property where the Co-operative Health Centre now stands.

The Origins of Stan Rands's Activism

What were the key factors that made Stan Rands a socialist, willing to support the social democratic CCF on common goals, but critical of the CCF government's cautious and incremental approach to social reform? As Lorne Brown points out in his introduction to the first edition, Rands was first influenced by the exigencies of the 1930s, from the rise of fascism in Europe which he saw at close hand while a Rhodes scholar at Oxford in the mid-1930s, to the Great Depression which he witnessed as a high school teacher in Alberta when he returned home.[9] In the 1930s, Rands seriously considered becoming a United Church minister, no doubt heavily influenced by the social gospel that was a powerful force within the CCF. However, it was his experiences during World War II that would radicalize his thinking.

In 1942, Rands moved to Winnipeg in order to become the assistant director of the University of Manitoba's Adult Education Office. He also moved into a 15-room co-operative house at 139 Roslyn Road that was filled by like-minded socialists and activists. Here, he came under the powerful influence of his new and charismatic boss, Watson Thomson, the director of adult education. Rands had likely met Thomson earlier, either in the United Kingdom where he was an activist and public intellectual, or after he moved to Canada to become a lecturer in the extension department of the University of Alberta from 1937–41.

Thomson was instrumental in assembling and mobilizing activists like Rands who would spend hours debating socialism in their Roslyn Road house. Thomson was the originator of the Prairie School for Social Advance, a leadership school for the more progressive-minded managers of civil society organizations, while Rands was a member of his Northern Plains Project, a study-action group whose goal was to establish and expand co-operatives in the Prairie Provinces. Some had linkages to the CCF in Manitoba but were distrusted as communists by the CCF party establishment who feared they were simply using, and in the process discrediting, the new party. When Thomson left Manitoba for Saskatchewan in 1944 to become the CCF government's new director of adult education, Stanley Knowles, a CCF member of Parliament from Winnipeg, sent a strongly-worded letter to Tommy Douglas about both Thomson and the Roslyn Road crowd. He was too late to prevent Douglas from hiring Thomson, but Knowles warned that he should never hire Rands, who had replaced Thomson as director of adult education at the University of Manitoba:

> My point in writing you is to remind you that the chap who succeeded W.T. in Manitoba is a very apt pupil of said W.T. In fact, it is one of those cases where the pupil outdistances the master... In any event, I feel I should give you a warning so that you may be in a position to prevent his being employed in Saskatchewan. I cannot make my warning too strong. It is very clear that we have a real struggle on our hands with these so-and-so's.[10]

This distrust was mutual. When Thomson was fired a little more than a year later by the Douglas government for his "propagandizing," he complained that the CCF in Saskatchewan had degenerated into a reformist social democratic party that had abandoned its mission to transform capitalist society. In his view, "the whole social democratic idea" should be "challenged" and "subjected to a radical evaluation" and, after his experience with "Social Democracy in action" in Saskatchewan, he concluded that

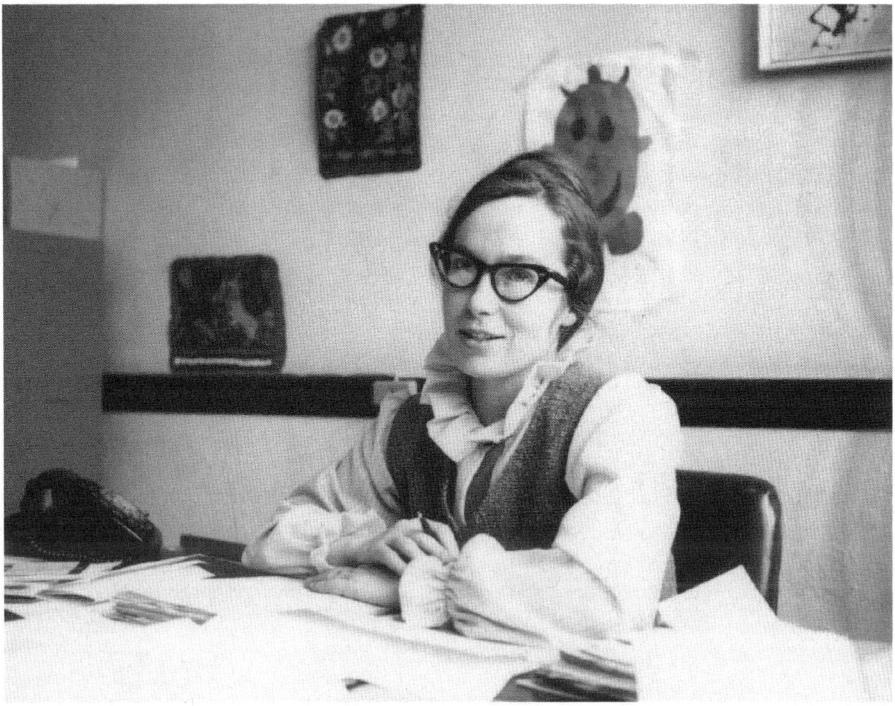

Mildred Kerr, Saskatoon Community Clinic social worker (Saskatoon Community Clinic photo #10-SK).

Thomson did not like it.[11] From the perspective of at least some within the CCF, Thomson and his Roslyn Road friends such as Rands, were "fellow travelers," the term used to describe communists who infiltrated the CCF in order to attack the party from within and discredit it from without.[12] Though there was no real evidence, much less proof, that Thomson was a member of the Communist Party, he became a victim of a growing anti-communist sentiment in Canada. In this also, Rands would follow in the footsteps of his mentor.

In 1945, Rands left Winnipeg for Ottawa to become a director of research and reports and coordinator of the distribution department at the National Film Board (NFB), where he would remain for five years. During this time, he was active on a civil liberties committee and spearheaded an effort to unionize workers at the NFB. Perhaps as a result of these activities and those he associated with in Ottawa, he was swept up in a mass firing at the NFB precipitated by the Cold War.[13]

Despite Knowles's earlier warning to Douglas, Rands was then hired by the CCF government in Saskatchewan, and he would remain in the province for the rest of his life. Rands spent a dozen years in the Department of Public Health, most of this time as Deputy Director of the Psychiatric Services Branch, the single largest unit within the provincial government. In this capacity, and as an active member of the Saskatchewan branch of the Canadian Mental Health Association, he worked to improve the plight of the mentally ill and to alter the negative stereotypes surrounding mental illness. In particular, he advocated in favour of closing down the province's two mental hospitals and shifting to a community-based model of mental care.[14]

As a senior civil servant within the department of government that was spearheading the implementation of medicare, Rands may have had a front row seat in the unfolding drama of the doctors' strike in July 1962, but only as a spectator.[15] The strike precipitated a province-wide movement by the most fervent supporters of medicare to fight back through the establishment of community clinics that would offer the services that striking doctors were refusing to provide.[16] More significantly, the community clinics offered an alternative approach to primary care, one in which doctors working in concert with other health professionals would provide a broader range of healthcare that included illness prevention and health promotion services. Rejecting the fee-for-service model defended so vigorously by organized medicine, clinic doctors were prepared to accept salaries and, free from having their remuneration tied to single transactions and patient visits, spend more time with individual patients.

By autumn 1962, Rands was being recruited from outside the government by William M. Harding to become the first permanent executive director of the Community Health Services Association (CHSA), the provincial umbrella organization for the community clinics.[17] The offer greatly appealed to Rands who had now concluded that he could do much more outside the government than inside.[18] And so he left.

In his new position, Rands had to deal with the deficiencies of the Saskatoon Agreement, and what he viewed as the tepid nature of the government's support for the community clinics, described in considerable detail in this book. In particular, the provincial government's refusal to replace fee-for-service with salaried remuneration for doctors meant that even community clinic doctors were forced by circumstance to accept fee-for-service payment despite their preference to work on salary.[19] Though Rands lobbied in favour of alternative remuneration for community clinic doctors for years, it would take the provincial government a decade after the doctors' strike to introduce global funding for community clinics.[20] By this time, however, the community clinics had shrunk in number after suffering years of difficulty, as Lawson and Thériault point out in their essay reprinted here.

To this day, the reform of primary care remains one of the most intractable pieces of the health care reform puzzle, and the potential for reform remains constrained by the Saskatoon Agreement. Primary health care continues to be dominated by doctors in private-for-profit professional practices and the majority of physicians in Canada continue to be remunerated through fee-for-service, limiting the time that doctors actually spend with their patients on either prevention or curative care. At the same time, some progress has been made since the 1960s. Contrary to Stan Rands's greatest fear, organized medicine has not undermined medicare despite the fact that most doctors remained committed to a for-profit fee-for-service model. Moreover, Rands urged the traditional family medicine model of primary care be replaced by a new model of interprofessional care involving nurses, social workers and others in addition to doctors, all working together in a group practice. Although this alternative model was considered by many to be radical in the early 1960s, it actually became the approach recommended by a majority of health experts in innumerable commissions and studies from the 1970s to the present.[21]

In fact, in recent years, a steadily rising percentage of doctors in Canada have accepted alternative payment and there is, at least among a certain number of younger doctors as well as women physicians, a growing interest in more collaborative practices.

What has not survived as well was Rands's argument concerning the advantages of salary. Indeed, there has been a growing consensus among the reformers that straight salary remuneration is almost as problematic as straight fee-for-service, and many have argued in favour of mixed or blended forms of payment for doctors.

Although decades have passed since the doctors' strike and the sharp debates on the direction of primary care reform, there remains a cleavage between those seeking more immediate and radical transformation and those pursuing a more incremental approach. In this sense, the debate of the 1960s that Stan Rands presents here remains relevant and important to the current debates concerning the reform of primary health care in Canada.

This is the 50th anniversary of the introduction of medicare in Saskatchewan. It is also the 50th anniversary of the establishment of community clinics in the province that posed a living and breathing alternative to the way in which we delivered—and continue to deliver—most primary health care in Canada. The fact that we have not been able to implement the second phase of medicare means that we need to better understand the history of medicare with all its compromises and tradeoffs.

Notes

1. Allan Blakeney quoted in Ann Silversides, *Conversations with Champions of Medicare* (Ottawa: Canadian Federation of Nurses Unions, 2007), 27.

2. C. David Naylor, *Private Practice, Public Payment: Canadian Medicine and the Politics of Health Insurance, 1911–1966* (Montreal and Kingston: McGill-Queen's University Press, 1986).

3. Carolyn H. Tuohy, "Single Payers, Multiple Systems: The Scope and Limits of Subnational Variation under a Federal Health Policy Framework," *Journal of Health Politics, Policy and Law* 34, no. 4 (2009): 453–96.

4. Stan Rands, "The CCF in Saskatchewan," in D.C. Kerr (ed.), *Western Canadian Politics: The Radical Tradition* (Edmonton: NeWest Institute for Western Canadian Studies, 1981), 58–64.

5. These were Douglas's reflections in 1982, quoted in Greg Marchildon, "The Douglas Legacy and the Future of Medicare," in Bruce Campbell and Greg Marchildon (eds.), *Medicare: Facts, Myths, Problems and Promise* (Toronto: James Lorimer and Company, 2007), 39–40.

6. Gordon S. Lawson, "The Road Not Taken: The 1945 Health Services Planning Commission Proposals and Physician Remuneration in Saskatchewan," *Canadian Bulletin of Medical History* 26, no. 2 (2009): 395–427.

7. Interview, Stuart Houston with author, January 13, 2010, and interview, Allan E. Blakeney with author, January 14, 2011.

8. Peter R. Sinclair, "The Saskatchewan CCF: Ascent to Power and the Decline of Socialism," *Canadian Historical Review* 54, no. 4 (1973): 419–33.

9. Curriculum vitae, biographies, job applications, promotion opportunities file, Box 48/66, Stan Rands Fonds, 85-80, University of Regina Archives (herafter SR Fonds): Rands was appointed Rhodes Scholar for Alberta in 1933 and then spent three years at Oxford University where he received a Diploma in Theology (1934) and a BA in politics, philosophy and economics (1936).

10. Knowles letter to Douglas, quoted in Ormond K. McKague, "'Socialist Education' in Saskatchewan, 1942–1948: A Study in Ideology and Bureaucracy" (PhD dissertation, University of Oregon, 1981), 264, and Michael R. Welton, "Conflicting Visions, Divergent Strategies: Watson Thomson and the Cold War Politics of Adult Education in Saskatchewan, 1944–6," *Labour/Le Travail* 18 (1986): 122.

11. McKague, "Socialist Education in Saskatchewan," 279.

12. Welton, "Conflicting Visions." Thomson's case contrasted with that of Dorise Nielsen, a CCF activist living near North Battleford, Saskatchewan, who joined the Communist Party of Canada in 1937 but did not disclose the fact of her membership until 1943. Faith Johnston, *A Great Restlessness: The Life and Politics of Dorise Nielsen* (Winnipeg: University of Manitoba Press, 2006).

13. Zoë Druick, *Projecting Canada: Government Policy and Documentary Film at the National Film Board* (Montreal and Kingston: McGill-Queen's University Press, 2007), 91.

14. Gregory P. Marchildon, "A House Divided: Deinstitutionalization, Medicare and the Canadian Mental Health Association in Saskatchewan, 1944–1964," *Histoire Sociale/Social History* 44, no. 88 (2011): 305–29.

15. The only evidence I could find of Rands's role at this time was his response to an Ontario doctor offering to come to Saskatchewan in the midst of the strike: letter, Rands to Dr. E.J.C. Otvos, 11 July 1962, Interest/Involvements/Issues file, Box 11, SR Fonds.

16. See Robin F. Badgley and Samuel Wolfe, *Doctors' Strike: Medical Care and Conflict in Saskatchewan* (Toronto: Macmillan of Canada, 1967), and Gregory P. Marchildon and Klaartje Schrijvers, "Physician Resistance and the Forging of Public Healthcare: A Comparative Analysis of the Doctors' Strikes in Canada and Belgium," *Medical History* 55, no. 2 (2011): 203–22.

17. Letter, W.M Harding (the temporary executive director of Community Health Services) to Rands, 29 Nov. 1962, CHSA Board of Directors file, SR Fonds.

18. Rands actually asked for a leave of absence and he waited some time before getting approval, one of the reasons he did not begin work as executive director for CHSA until January 8, 1963. His leave of absence was cancelled five years later: Letters: Rands to F.S. Lawson, 21 Dec. 1962, and J.G. Clarkson to Rands, 20 Dec. 1965, Box 48/66, SR Fonds.

19. Samuel Wolfe, "Saskatchewan's Community Clinics," *Canadian Medical Association Journal* 91 (1964): 225–29.

20. The CHSA Regina Newsletter, Nov. 1972, Box 12, 89-70, SR Fonds.

21. Roy Romanow, *Building on Values: The Future of Health Care in Canada, Final Report* (Saskatoon: Commission on the Future of Health Care in Canada, 2002). Brian Hutchison, Jean-Frederic Levesque, Erin Strumpf and Natalie Coyle, "Primary Health Care in Canada: Systems in Motion," *Milbank Quarterly* 89, no. 2 (2011): 256–88.

Foreword to the 1994 Edition: Stan Rands: A Hidden Hero of Medicare

Benjamin G. Smillie

When a writer faces the task of fleshing out a personality who played a significant role in a major historical event, the task is made easier if that person has had a high political profile. But Stan Rands's accomplishments usually appear as footnotes. His name pops up time and again in the minutes of community clinic meetings—particularly in 1962, when Saskatchewan became the first province in Canada to establish prepaid medical care—but it is not trumpeted at political rallies or in newspaper headlines. Nine years after his death and 33 years after the medicare crisis, Stan Rands remains an elusive person. Even in this book, which relates and encompasses the major work of his life, he never talks about his own accomplishments.

While there are disadvantages in searching out the life of a retiring personality, there are also advantages. As I began to call on Stan's friends, I found many people who wanted to help with the manuscript—many more than I could possibly use, and some of them had held important positions in the establishing of medicare in Saskatchewan. Seeing the obvious admiration people still held for Stan Rands, the biographical task became a pleasure. Unfortunately, Dr. Ed Mahood and Dr. Sam Wolfe, who gave me valuable insights into Stan's life, have died since I interviewed them.

Everyone agrees that Stan was a gracious man. Through the often intractable community of the militant left in Canada, Stan Rands rode with consideration and care for the women and men he worked with, often giving financial help to those in need, with no expectation of receiving anything in return. No doubt he drew strength from his wife, Doris, as she drew strength from him.

As Doris Rands describes it, she met Stan "through a lucky accident" in 1943, when she was teaching in Russell, Manitoba:

> His boss, Watson Thomson, had been invited to lead an adult education seminar in Russell, and my boss, the school principal, was to meet his train and take him to dinner. Watson couldn't come so sent his assistant, Stan, and my boss couldn't meet the train so sent me.[1]

What Doris calls a "lucky accident" Jungians would describe as synchronicity, and Christians as providence. However it happened, they made a remarkable team. Bea Harding, active in the community clinics that seemed to spring up overnight in 1962, recalls that the Randses were constantly befriending people who showed up on their doorstep flat broke. "They got nothing in return, but they never complained."[2] Indeed, Stan Rands, who calmly stood with Doris in the eye of the storm, is one of the true heroes of Saskatchewan medicare, and therefore a national hero of Canada.

Medicare in Canada makes us distinctive and proud. The United States, a far wealthier country, has a plan that takes care of the aged, but the majority of the population remains without benefits. In 1965 it was estimated that only 2.5% of the American population "received comprehensive health services from prepaid medical groups."[3] In Canada, by contrast, the Medical Care Act, providing Canadians with universal coverage, became law in 1966.

Martha Livingston, one of Stan Rands's graduate students at the University of Regina and now a professor of Community Health in the United States, writes of Rands's impact on an American audience:

> ... any time I talk to progressive Canadian health care researchers and activists, Stan is remembered with great respect and fondness. Stan was received as a guest of honour at the 1978 national conference of the Medical Committee for Human Rights in Philadelphia, where he enthralled his audience of progressive American doctors and health professionals.[4]

What is there in Saskatchewan that made us hang tough in 1962 when universal medicare was established? The plan has been emulated throughout the country and abroad, but for a time it seemed it might not happen at all. There is a familiar chant you hear at New Democratic Party rallies, naming the patron saints of medicare: Tommy Douglas and Woodrow Lloyd, with a nod to some of the national big names such as Justice Emmet Hall and, more recently, Monique Bégin. But if you read the story of medicare only through the feats of these people you will get a "laundered" version of history.[5] The real heroes of medicare in Saskatchewan were the hard-line socialists who put iron into the political will of the CCF-NDP and kept them from caving in to the international medical lobby.

As Stand Rands explains in this book, the medicare crisis in Saskatchewan was caused not by the toughness of the CCF government in 1962, nor by the establishment of the Medical Care Insurance Commission, nor by the diplomatic skills of Lord Stephen Taylor which brought about the end of the doctors' strike and the establishment of medicare in the province. No, the threat to the medical establishment was the growth of community health clinics, which sprang up like mushrooms in the weeks after the doctors went on strike on July 1, 1962. As soon as it became clear that certain doctors were willing to work as salaried employees of community clinic boards, the medical establishment as a whole trembled.

The power of the left in Canadian politics has always been its intelligent understanding of underlying issues, and a resolution not to compromise. In Saskatchewan, the left has always had influence beyond its numerical strength. An unfortunate side effect of this is that socialists have a way of becoming fractious, partly because of the stress of often being the lone voice in opposition, but also because—and perhaps this is a consequence of the former—they tend to be hard on one another in personal relationships. Stan Rands became a sort of talisman for the left, providing gracious and imaginative leadership to break out of what could have become an ideological impasse. Dennis Gruending, author of an early history of the Saskatoon Community Clinic, interviewed Stan in 1973:

> ... with the unassuming graciousness that was his trademark, Stan patiently answered all of my questions. Later I met Doris, and saw

> that she and Stan shared similar qualities of erudition and quiet determination, which coexisted with their passionate belief in progressive causes.[6]

Jack Shapiro, a long-time activist on the left, characterizes Stan Rands as a man who "had the loveliest way of looking at everything. He had a great mind and a marvellous sense of humour."[7]

He used that great mind, his remarkable intellectual capacity, for the public good. He was a top-flight scholar, but he was not content to spend his life within the sheltered walls of academia. He was an educator who could not stay away from the hurly-burly of politics—what the Italian Marxist Antonio Gramsci would call an "organic intellectual," one whose knowledge concentrates on creating a praxis between theory and application. For Gramsci, knowledge is based not on abstract reason but on common sense. Only as the intellectual engages in real-life issues do the theories become purified.[8]

Ken Collier, a professor of social work at the University of Regina, shows how Stan Rands personifies the organic intellectual. He describes a trip he took with Stan in 1965:

> ... I drove Stan to Eston, north of Swift Current, for an evening meeting. Although exhausted, he was to present complex financial and other materials to a newly elected clinic board. Just out of Regina, he put a pillow against the car window, and went immediately to sleep. We stopped for fuel in Swift Current. Only when we turned west toward Eston did Stan awake, apparently refreshed, [he] skimmed through a file of notes, ate supper in Eston over more notes, and he marched into that meeting to deliver a crisp, information-laden, but digestible address.[9]

One of the issues that taxed Stan Rands's patience and frustrated his sense of fair play was the harassment community clinic doctors had to undergo when seeking hospital privileges. "Few things are more damaging to morale," he wrote, "than to be ready for a battle in which you know you are right, but to have your hands tied behind your back."[10]

The harassment over hospital privileges for community clinic doctors was contrary to the Saskatoon Agreement of 1962, which provided that:

> There must be no discrimination against any doctor in whatsoever way he [*sic*] practices. In particular there must be no discrimination against any doctor in the matter of hospital privileges and attachments... .[11]

The breaking of the Agreement was clear in a case involving the right of Dr. Rene Gold to have hospital privileges in Saskatoon City Hospital. After many delays Dr. Gold's case was heard by the Royal Commission, which had been set up under Justice Mervyn Woods to investigate such problems. Justice Woods's judgement, as Dr. Gold remembers it, "detected evidence of political bias against community clinic doctors as a whole":

> In my case, it said the hospital had decided with an incomplete knowledge of the facts and that I had reasons for supposing that the decision to deny me privileges had been motivated by political considerations.

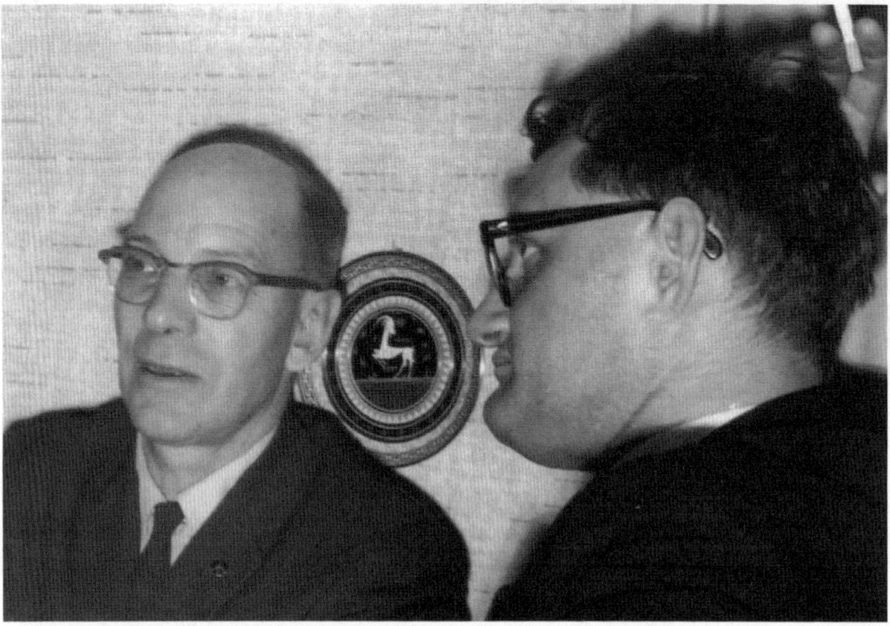

Stan Rands and Dr. René Gold, n.d. (Saskatoon Community Clinic Photo #5-SK).

> Given this judicial hint, the city hospital reconsidered the question of my hospital privileges and they were finally granted to me. In the course of this reconsideration, it came out that the Medical Advisory Committee had concealed all my good references from the Hospital Board and revealed only the bad ones.[12]

The frustration this episode represented is reflected again and again in the civilized anger that is sometimes evident in this book. Stan Rands's ability to be flexible with those he worked with, however, more often dampened anger than fuelled it. For example, it has often been difficult in Saskatchewan to get farmers and labour to work together. It is rather remarkable that when Stan was Executive Secretary of the Community Health Services Association in the 1960s, the first president was Clarence Lyons and the second was Roy Atkinson. Lyons, a former president of the Saskatchewan Federation of Labour, recalls that Rands was "a good friend of labour, and was used frequently by us in arbitration hearings because he had the ability to see fair solutions after tough bargaining."[13] Roy Atkinson was president of the National Farmers Union and the most prominent farmer in the province.

Another way in which Stan Rands showed flexibility was his recognition, in the face of the intransigence of the medical-political lobby on the fee-for-service issue, that it was important to develop an alternative. He saw the possibility of developing within community clinics a method of providing health care delivery on a "global budget." David Penman, a British doctor with an intimate knowledge of the National Health Service in that country, was brought into the Department of Health when the NDP was returned to power in 1971. He became the main architect of a plan to give the community clinics the right to establish alternative systems of financing. He characterized Stan Rands as "a strong opponent of a fee-for-service system":

> ... he had hoped that with the return of the province to an NDP administration in 1971 that steps toward a salaried method of payment for health would be introduced in Saskatchewan; in this he was disappointed. Stan pushed, in common with others, for the introduction of global budgeting for community clinics; this was successful and permitted community clinics to examine alternative and innovative approaches to health care for their members.[14]

In Stan Rands's view the Saskatoon Agreement called on the CCF government through the establishment of a Medical Care Insurance Commission (MCIC) to establish clinics and encourage the recruitment of doctors to work for salaries. Although he writes without rancour, Stan insists that the MCIC became intimidated by the anti-medicare lobby and did not do enough to support doctors who were working for community clinics. They listened instead to the doctors' lobby, some of whom were out to destroy prepaid medicare. Dr. Orville Hjertaas, the director of the Prince Albert Community Clinic and a member of the first Medical Care Insurance Commission appointed by the government in 1962, responds that, after the Saskatoon Agreement the MCIC was reduced to being a paying agency for doctors. To begin with, the MCIC paid the money to the doctors' insurance brokers, Medical Services Incorporated (MSI), because the doctors didn't want to touch the government's tainted money. But after a short time doctors were billing the MCIC directly so that they could get their money faster. The real political power, according to Dr. Hjertaas, lay in the hospital boards, who were hand-in-glove with the Saskatchewan Medical Association. He recalls, in fact, that in the middle of the doctors' strike a meeting of the medical staff of the Prince Albert hospital was held in the office of one of the leaders of the Keep Our Doctors Committee. He goes on to explain that hospital boards, which were supposed to be servants of the public and dispensers of public money, acted instead as the doctors's' agents.[15]

Roy Atkinson, then president of the National Farmers Union and the second president of the Community Health Services Association, believes that the doctors were at the end of their tether when they signed the Saskatoon Agreement on July 23, 1962. They were out of money and they had used up their holiday time. "I sat outside the cabinet room in the Legislative Building for two days, telling them not to settle," Atkinson recalls. "But we were eventually ushered into the cabinet room and told the strike was over and we should withdraw our pressure and acquiesce to the demands of the doctors."[16] Ed Mahood, first chairperson of the Saskatoon Community Health Clinic Board, agrees that the government need not have settled with the doctors so quickly, and would in fact have been able to develop a system in which doctors worked on salary under a community clinic board as an option.[17]

But there were others active in the CCF who maintain that Woodrow Lloyd and his embattled government could not have done more than they did. Jack Shapiro saw the terrible wrath of the doctors and the Keep Our Doctors Committee on May 3, 1962, when Woodrow Lloyd walked into the Trianon Ballroom in Regina to address them. Shapiro says he had never seen "a public figure take such abuse and vilification and walk away with dignity." The left thinks the community clinics were the instruments of a counter force that brought the doctors to end their strike, Shapiro says, but if the clinics were as influential as claimed, how is it that they have given such a

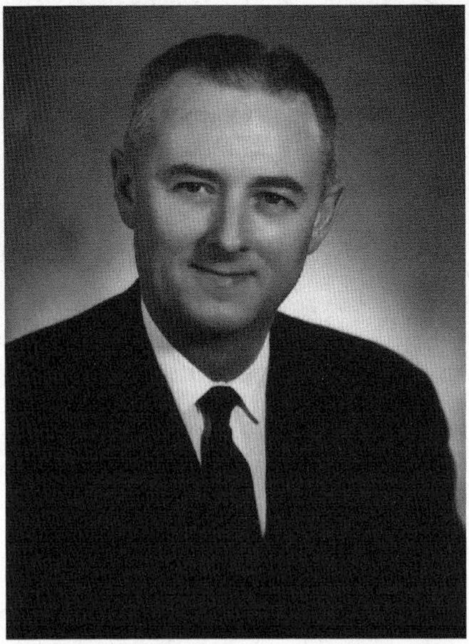

C.A. "Smokey" Robson, n.d. (Saskatoon Community Clinic photo #18-SK).

lacklustre performance in subsequent health care delivery? He concludes that perhaps the government was aware that community clinics were not as strong as their own propaganda maintained.[18] George Taylor, a distinguished Saskatoon labour lawyer who provided liaison between the government and the chief negotiator, Lord Stephen Taylor, agrees with Jack Shapiro that the government did the best they could. Many of the cabinet and the public were tired of the battle and wanted to bring political peace to the province.[19]

Dr. Margaret Mahood, comparing the scene in 1962 to 1993, says that we should get over the doctor-bashing and recognize that they no longer enjoy the power they once had.[20] No doubt the debate will continue with the advantage of hindsight, but Stan Rands would not want us to rethresh old straw.

The person who perhaps can give the best overview of community health clinics in Saskatchewan is C.A. "Smokey" Robson, who joined the board of the Community Clinic in Saskatoon in 1963.[a] He has been a facility planner for the community clinics, he has served as chairperson of the board of the Saskatoon Community Clinic, and in 1971 was appointed its Administrator. He retired from that position in 1983, but remains a vigorous secretary of the Community Health Co-operative Federation, an umbrella organization that looks into joint planning for the community clinics in the province.

I felt Smokey was the best person to fill in the gaps in Stan Rands's story of the community clinic movement. Stan writes, for example, that in March 1963, "almost 15,000 families, representing approximately 50,000 people, in 36 areas of the province [had] joined the community clinic movement," and that "eight associations [had] purchased or built clinic premises" and "$325,000 [had] been raised through memberships, donations, and loans of various kinds." Yet today there are only five clinics in the province: Prince Albert, Regina, Saskatoon, and two smaller ones in Lloydminster and Wynyard. How did this come about?

Smokey traces the fallout through Stan's correspondence, which is now filed in the Provincial Archives in Saskatoon under "Community Health Co-operative Federation." Stan's passionate support for community clinics shows up best in his letters, and he

[a] Cecil A. "Smokey" Robson passed away in 2010. After he retired as Administrator of the Saskatoon Community Clinic, he also served as president of this clinic's foundation as well as chair of the clinic board for two additional terms: see John Bury, Betsy Bury, Stan Rice, Ingrid Larson, Judy Martin and Patrick Lapointe, "C.A. 'Smokey' Robson: A Useful Life," *Focus* 46, no. 1 (2010): 6–7.

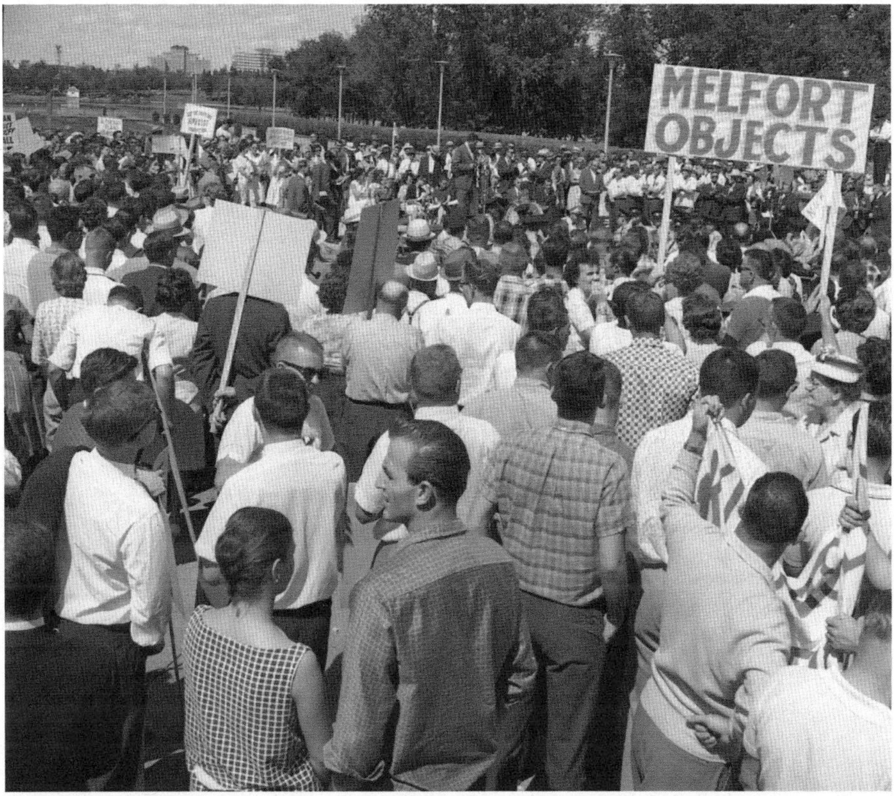

The Melfort contingent at the Keep Our Doctors Rally, July 11, 1962 (SAB R-PS62-229, Photographic Services Series, Photo #23).

kept up his correspondence with people on clinic boards around the province long after the physical facility in a particular area had disappeared. Smokey was able to give me a thumbnail sketch of what happened to the clinics that closed. In each case, there was a familiar pattern of harassment.

The Eston clinic had no problem getting a physician. The problem was the hospital, whose board was not sympathetic to the clinic. The other doctors in Eston followed a policy of keeping the hospital beds filled with their own patients. This effectively denied the clinic doctor access to the local hospital. If he was to have a full practice, he had to admit his patients to the hospital in Brock, 28 kilometres away. The Eston group eventually gave up on their clinic around 1975.

The Biggar association operated a community clinic for many years, but it would not allow extra billing, which their doctors demanded, when the practice became common in the mid-1980s. Clinic doctors responded by setting up their own clinic in 1985. The association still owns the building, but it has been unsuccessful in securing a doctor to work in it. The premises are currently rented to a law firm.[b]

The Melfort clinic recruited four physicians, but they were all denied hospital

[b] The Biggar association continues to rent its space and donates the proceeds to health-related charitable organizations (personal communication with Jim Kerr, president of the Biggar Community Clinic, July 2010).

privileges, so the operation dispersed. The pattern was much the same in Estevan, Moose Jaw, Nipawin, Weyburn, Radville, Kamsack, Kindersley, and Kinistino. North Battleford, with a membership of some 700 families, recruited two doctors and managed to stay in operation until 1963, but their constant struggle for survival eventually forced them into bankruptcy.

Two rural communities in which community clinics have survived are Wynyard and Lloydminster, each with around 300 members.[c] The Lloydminster clinic employs three doctors, and for the past five years has been incorporated under the co-operative act, so the members are actually shareholders.[d] The precarious success of the Wynyard clinic is owing largely to Sharon Armstrong, a charismatic school teacher who serves as chairperson of the clinic board as well as mayor of the town. Of the three community clinics that are thriving, Prince Albert has about 4,500 members, while Saskatoon and Regina have about 6,000 each.[e]

Smokey's assessment of the situation is an eloquent reminder that, when the legitimacy of health care services is dependent on the number of doctors you have, then doctors remain the gatekeepers of health. This model has come under heavy criticism lately, and clinics are trying to promote the wellness model as an alternative. Unfortunately, as long as doctors are *de facto* in charge, privilege will continue to determine health policy.

For my own part, I was a second-string player in the medicare drama, one member of a large committee that established Citizens in Defense of Medicare in 1962. I was also chairperson of a small committee in 1962 which started Citizens for a Free Press in Saskatoon. We wanted the Saskatoon *StarPhoenix* to publish the letters in favour of

[c] The Lloydminster clinic is in the process of selling its assets and a meeting to dissolve the co-operative is forthcoming (personal communication with Joe Holden, vice-president of the Lloydminster Community Clinic, October 2011).

[d] Since 1983, community clinics have been able to incorporate under the Co-operatives Act. Before that time, there were three pieces of legislation concerning co-operatives, but none were appropriate for the delivery of health care services and so clinics registered under the Mutual Medical and Hospital Benefit Association Act. The three distinct co-operative acts were replaced with a single piece of legislation for all co-operatives in 1983, and this features a chapter specifically on community clinics: see *The Co-operatives Act, 1996* (Regina: Queen's Printer, 1996). The Prince Albert, Regina and Saskatoon Community Clinics are now incorporated as co-operatives. However, members do not purchase shares in community clinics in Saskatchewan. This differs from other forms of co-operatives such as worker co-operatives or commercially oriented consumer co-operatives. Instead, individuals may choose to become members by paying a one-time membership fee. Obtaining a membership allows individuals to run for the board of directors, serve on committees, and receive clinic newsletters, if available.

[e] In its 2010/2011 fiscal year, the Saskatoon clinic provided health care services to 12,676 individuals and had an annual operating budget of $11.3 million: see Community Health Services Association (Saskatoon) Ltd, *Saskatoon Community Clinic 2010/2011 Year in Review*. Over the same period, the Regina clinic provided services to 5,280 individuals (*Regina Community Clinic Statistics for Saskatchewan Health*, March 31, 2011) and had an operating budget of $3.6 million (personal communication with Mary Flynn, administrator of the Regina Community Clinic, October 2011). The Prince Albert Clinic had an annual budget of $6.5 million over the 2010/2011 fiscal year (Co-operative Health Centre Prince Albert, *49th Annual Meeting Report*, 2011). The number of discrete patient visits was not available from this clinic. No data from the Wynyard clinic were available.

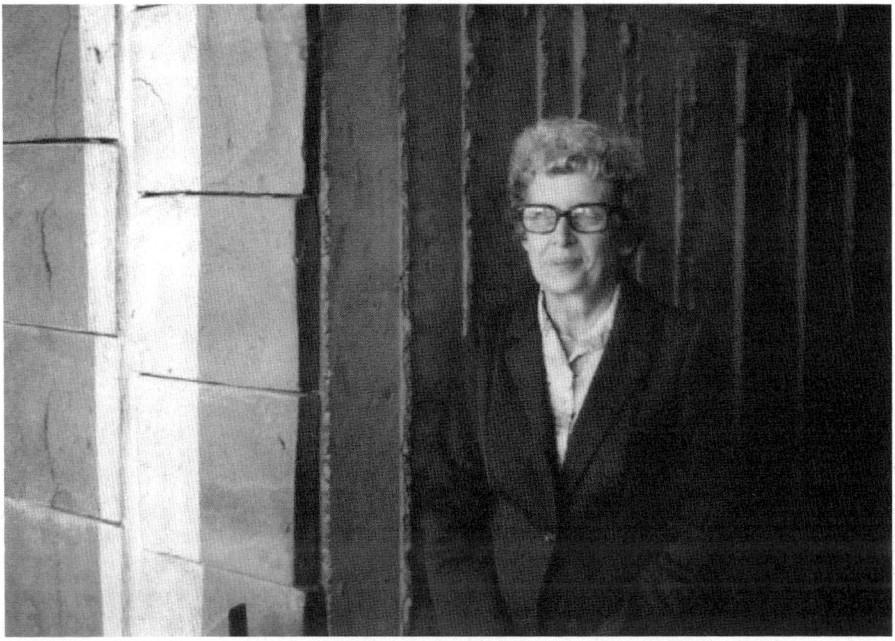

Grete Lebeau, the first Member Relations Officer of the Saskatoon Community Clinic (Saskatoon Community Clinic, photo # 6-SK).

medicare which they were receiving but not printing. We finally got through to Saskatoon citizens by buying advertising space in the *StarPhoenix* and printing the letters the newspaper had rejected. The committee dissolved after two months when the *StarPhoenix* started to publish our letters.[21]

The medicare crisis impinged on our family life as well. In 1962 my wife, Adele, was pregnant with our youngest daughter, and our doctor, Rene Gold, was being denied hospital privileges. Everything turned out in the end, but in hindsight it is exceedingly strange that a competent and fully qualified physician should be denied access to a publicly owned hospital.

While I knew Stan Rands through his leadership during the medicare crisis, I have found out more about him through his friends. Grete Lebeau, the first Member Relations Officer of the Saskatoon Community Clinic, remembers that she and her husband, George, "first met Stanley Rands in late 1939 in the city of Edmonton. We met through a mutual friend, Watson Thomson. At that time in history Stan was a graduate in theology and about to become an ordained minister of the United Church of Canada."[22]

I was unaware that Stan Rands had considered going into the ministry of the United Church. Too frequently, the only person in ministry who is mentioned in the crisis is Father Atholl Murray of Wilcox, with his incendiary statements on behalf of the Keep our Doctors Committee. "We must get off the fence and make our views known," he declared. "This thing may break out into violence and bloodshed any day now, and God help us if it doesn't."[23] By contrast, the United Church General Council, meeting in Edmonton in 1960, supported a plan of universal prepaid medical care.[24] In 1962 the Saskatchewan Conference of the United Church endorsed the General

Council statement and supported the Saskatchewan government's action to introduce prepaid medical care.

Gregory Vlastos (1907–1991), a United Church minister and a founder of the Fellowship for a Christian Social Order, once prayed, "Give us the patience of those who understand, and the impatience of those who love."[25] That would be my epitaph for Stan Rands: he had the patience of one who understood, and the impatience of one who loved.

He kept the faith.

Notes

A United Church minister and political activist for most of his life, Ben Smillie died in Saskatoon on May 31, 2011, at the age of 87. He was the author of six books including *Beyond the Social Gospel* and *Christian Ethics in a Pluralistic Society*. Obituary by Philip Fine in *Globe and Mail*, June 15, 2011.

1. Doris Rands, fax to B.G. Smillie, Vancouver, April 11, 1993.

2. Bea Harding, interview with B.G. Smillie, Regina, March 12, 1993.

3. Samuel Wolfe and Robin F. Badgley, *The Family Doctor* (Toronto: Macmillan of Canada, 1973), 14.

4. Martha Livingston, fax to B.G. Smillie, Old Westbury, New York, April 7, 1993.

5. Daniel Drache, "Rediscovering Canadian Political Economy," in Wallace Clement and Daniel Drache, *A Practical Guide to Canadian Political Economy* (Toronto: James Lorimer, 1978), 28–32. Political economist Drache says that many of his colleagues, analyzing the structures of capitalism, are "launderers"—they wash out the class conflict. Historians, too, can be launderers when they take as given the official interpretation of events.

6. Dennis Gruending, fax to B.G. Smillie, Ottawa, April 13, 1993. Dennis is the author of *The First Ten Years* (Saskatoon Community Clinic, 1973), as well as biographies of Justice Emmet Hall and Allan Blakeney.

7. Jack Shapiro, interview with B.G. Smillie, Saskatoon, March 30, 1993. Before coming to Saskatchewan Shapiro had been a member of the Workers Education Association in Toronto, an educational union under contract to the United Auto Workers. He lost his job when Walter Reuther, a red-baiting American union leader, became president of the UAW.

8. Antonio Gramsci, *Selections from the Prison Notebooks of Antonio Gramsci*, Quinton Hoare and Geoffrey Nowell Smith (eds. and trans.) (New York: International Publishers, 1971), 330.

9. Ken Collier, fax to B.G. Smillie, Saskatoon, April 16, 1993. Collier was the administrator of the Battleford Community Clinic in 1964. The clinic had a sporadic life between 1962 and 1964 but eventually had to close owing to lack of funds.

10. See amended manuscript, page 125, Rands private papers, University of Regina Archives.

11. *Saskatoon Agreement: Memorandum of Agreement, Government of the Province of Saskatchewan and the College of Physicians and Surgeons of Saskatchewan*, 4.

12. Dr. Rene Gold, fax to B.G. Smillie, Montreal, April 19, 1993.

13. Clarence Lyons, interview with B.G. Smillie, Saskatoon, April 14, 1993.

14. Dr. David Penman, fax to B.G. Smillie, Ottawa, April 13, 1993.

15. Dr. Orville Hjertaas, interview with B.G. Smillie, Prince Albert, March 30, 1993.

16. Roy Atkinson, interview with B.G. Smillie, Saskatoon, March 23, 1993.

17. Dr. Margaret Mahood and Dr. Ed Mahood, interview with B.G. Smillie, Saskatoon, March

18, 1993. Margaret Mahood was a psychiatrist with the Saskatoon Community Clinic medical staff who agreed to treat patients during the doctors' strike as salaried employees working under the MCIC. Ed Mahood was a pioneer of the community clinic movement in Saskatchewan and twice chairperson of the Community Health Services (Saskatoon) Association. Both Margaret and Ed speak with enthusiasm of the socialist study group in Regina in the 1940s and 1950s. The group included Hub and Elsie Elkin, Bill and Bea Harding, Stan and Doris Rands, Jack and Juliette Shapiro, Walter and Ruth Smishek, Edith and David Smith, Murray Thompson, and Len and Norma Wallace. After 1955 there was less discussion and more action as a younger generation joined them. This led to the nucleus of the left who formed the Waffle in the 1970s. Martha Livingston remembers the "halcyon days of the Saskatchewan Waffle" (Livingston, *op cit.*).

18. Jack Shapiro interview.

19. George Taylor, interview with B.G. Smillie, Saskatoon, April 5, 1993. Taylor had perhaps the clearest picture of what was going on between the three main groups in the crisis: the government, the doctors, and the negotiator.

20. Mahood interview.

21. Citizens for a Free Press in Saskatoon included Doug Cherry, a professor of English at the University of Saskatchewan, later Dean of Arts and Science, who wrote most of our press releases; Jim Naylor, a biology professor, treasurer, who was constantly amazed at the large amounts of money coming into our postal box; Stuart Thiessen, executive secretary of the National Farmers Union; and Benjamin G. Smillie, at that time a campus chaplain.

22. Grete Lebeau, letter to B.G. Smillie, White Rock, BC, March 31, 1993.

23. Robin F. Badgley and Samuel Wolfe, *Doctors' Strike: Medical Care and Conflict in Saskatchewan* (Toronto: Macmillan of Canada, 1967), 65.

24. Record of Proceedings of the Nineteenth General Council of the United Church of Canada (Edmonton: n.p., 1960), 101.

25. Gregory Vlastos, "For Firmness," in John W. Doberstein (ed.), *Minister's Prayer Book* (Philadelphia: Fortress Press, 1959), 165–66.

Introduction to the 1994 Edition: Engaged in the Work of the World

Lorne A. Brown

In this book Stan Rands depicts the long, often bitter struggle to establish universal access to medical care as a *right*, the same as the right to attend a publicly funded school system. He also discusses the equally long and not always successful struggle to assert democratic control over publicly funded medical care.

Stan's discussion of the issues is centred mainly on Saskatchewan, where he was in the front lines of the battle and provided superb leadership over many years. But the same battle was joined throughout North America and much of the world, and medical issues comprised only one of many fronts in a worldwide class and ideological struggle which accelerated in the 1930s and which has influenced virtually all economic and political debate since World War II.

Stanley Rands was born at Fort Macleod, Alberta, in 1909. He attended public and high school in Fort Macleod, then went on to complete an arts degree at the University of Alberta, with classes in psychology as well as theology classes from St Stephen's College, a United Church theological college affiliated with the University of Alberta. An academic gold medalist and a Rhodes scholar, Stan began his studies at Oxford in 1933, the worst year of the Great Depression. Much of the world was polarizing on a right-left axis. That same year, Hitler seized power in Germany, Japanese militarists were carrying on a war of aggression against China, and fascist and militarist movements were on the rise in many other countries. Events in Spain would lead in a few years to the Spanish Civil War, the fiercest left-right conflict in Europe before the outbreak of World War II.

At Oxford, Stan Rands was exposed to many of the debates then raging in intellectual circles. The left was on the rise not only among the working class but also among a growing minority of the intelligentsia. Socialist, communist, and labour movements were flourishing across Europe. In the United States, Franklin Roosevelt was beginning his New Deal. In Canada, the Co-operative Commonwealth Federation (CCF) issued its famous Regina Manifesto in 1933.

It was in this context that Stan Rands returned from Oxford to Alberta, where he completed his education and began teaching in 1937. Much of the prairies were struggling with conflicting versions of prairie populism, although by then "Bible Bill" Aberhart's Social Credit movement had formed the provincial government and the once powerful United Farmers of Alberta had been virtually destroyed. Their successor, the CCF, would never be a significant force in Alberta politics.

Stan soon moved to Winnipeg, where he worked in adult education and for the National Film Board, which was coming into its own during the war years. In 1943, he married Doris Fraser, a Manitoba schoolteacher, and together they took up the educational and political work which was to engage them for the rest of their lives. They lived first in a Winnipeg co-operative, a commune not of people who had withdrawn from society but of people who were engaged fully in the work of the world. They were in many respects on the cutting edge of various struggles for social change, and some of them paid a steep personal price for it during the Cold War.

One commune member was Watson Thomson, the renowned adult educator who attempted to implement a "pedagogy of liberation" which would enable people to take power into their own hands. He worked for the first CCF government in Saskatchewan until he was forced out because of his radical views.[1] Another was Berry Richards who became CCF MLA for Flin Flon, and was then expelled from the party because of his views on the Cold War. Richards was later active in the politics of northern Saskatchewan.

Stan Rands was also a victim of the Cold War.[2] In 1945, he and Doris had moved to Ottawa, where Stan became director of research and program co-ordinator for the distribution department of the National Film Board. It was an exciting time to be at the NFB, which was then under the brilliant leadership of John Grierson. During their years in Ottawa, Stan and Doris were active in political study groups, adult education, and civil liberties and trade union activities with the Civil Service Association. That came to an end in 1950 when Stan, along with Grierson and scores of others, fell victim to the McCarthyism which emasculated the NFB and other agencies, in the process destroying the careers of some of the most imaginative civil servants in Ottawa.

It was this experience which brought Stan to Regina in the fall of 1950. In the provincial capital he worked in health education under the auspices of the Provincial Health Department, later becoming Deputy Director of Psychiatric Services for the province. He continued his political activities, but in a much more progressive environment. It was political education, agitation, and organization in the health care field that most interested him. His leading role in the medicare crisis and in the struggle to establish community clinics was a natural outgrowth of this work.

Stan remained a health care activist for the rest of his life. In his view, health care issues interlocked with many others, so it was only natural for him to become involved in civil liberties, aboriginal rights, peace, and labour activities. He was also a leading activist in the Waffle movement of the 1970s. His unique and compassionate voice will long be an inspiration to others.

In this book Stan reveals his depth of knowledge of not only the historical struggles of the movement for social medicine but also of how it relates to the broader struggle for social emancipation in Saskatchewan, Canada, and on the international scene.

Chapter 1 examines the historical political economy of Saskatchewan and the conflict between social movements and organized medicine over the delivery of medical services in the province. This would pit the farm and labour movements and the State Hospital and Medical League against the Canadian Medical Association and their provincial supporters. The first tentative steps toward medicare by the CCF governments after 1944 are described as a prelude to the great struggle of 1962.

Chapter 2 is a superb treatment of the historical success of the Canadian Medical

Association and the American Medical Association to establish a powerful monopoly over medical procedures and the delivery of medical services throughout this continent. They would control almost the entire ideological approach to medicine, and Stan provides us with important insights as to how their interests overlapped with the interests of the insurance industry and the corporate world in general. The latest example of this is the fate of President Clinton's attempt to institute a limited universal medicare plan in the United States.

The analysis of the attempt to implement medicare in Saskatchewan and the Saskatoon Agreement in 1962 illustrates that the battle with the doctors was inevitable, as it grew out of the struggles of the past. Attempts to build viable community clinics and move away from the fee-for-service system further illustrates the tremendous power of organized medicine and their allies. Through Chapters 5 to 8, Stan discusses how the clinic movement was frustrated at every turn by recruiting problems, financial problems, denial of hospital privileges, and the ostracism of clinic doctors. The sabotage by organized medicine coupled with a lack of support from the provincial government made the community clinic movement a pale shadow of what it might have been.

In the last two chapters Stan reminds us of the progressive yet limited relationship of the labour movement to the medical system. He reiterates the history of the long struggle and reminds us that the job is only half done. This is typical of Stan, who was never one to be satisfied with half measures.

Notes

1. Michael R. Welton, "Conflicting Visions, Divergent Strategies: Watson Thomson and the Cold War Politics of Adult Education in Saskatchewan, 1944–6," *Labour/Le Travail* (Fall 1986).

2. Len Scher, "Lives on the Cutting Room Floor"; interview with Doris Rands, *The Un-Canadians: True Stories of the Blacklist Era* (Toronto, Lester Publishing Ltd, 1992).

Chapter 1
The Roots of the Community Clinic Movement

People from outside the province often express surprise at the suddenness with which community clinics sprang up across Saskatchewan after the Medical Care Insurance Act was passed in 1961. They see it as a kind of mushroom growth that happened almost overnight, largely in reaction to the medicare crisis. While it is true that the movement was closely linked to the bitter politics of the time, and that the move to organize was a direct response to that crisis, community clinics were also a result of the ideas and experiences of Saskatchewan people over 60 years.

Between 1900 and 1921, the population of rural Saskatchewan increased sevenfold as national policy encouraged immigration and settlement. The rural population grew from 86,000 in 1901 to 630,000 in 1921.[1] This precipitous growth created many health problems, as new settlements often had inadequate sanitary facilities, and contagious diseases spread quickly. The need to improve living conditions in rural areas led in 1909 to the Rural Municipalities Act which, as well as establishing areas of jurisdiction in the province, made the municipality accountable for the care of needy persons within its boundaries. Revenues for this purpose were to be raised through a general land tax,[2] with municipal councils responsible for improving the living conditions of their populations.

Their success or failure depended on the local farm economy. Municipalities with a low indigent population could generally cover the costs of relief, but municipal councils had no control over the economy: the price of wheat was set by provincial grain buyers. In poorer municipalities, where large numbers of farm families were unable to pay for food, shelter, or medical care, living conditions did not improve.

Because poorer areas often could not afford to pay their doctors, many physicians moved to wealthier municipalities or to the cities. In 1911 there was one doctor for every 1,298 people in the province, and the majority practised in or around urban areas which were largely inaccessible to rural people.[3] In response, and without legislative authority, some rural municipalities began offering retainer fees to their doctors. In 1914, for example, the RM of Sarnia offered its doctor $1,500 as an annual retainer.[4] The doctor, in return, was to provide free medical care to indigent persons in the area. Patients who could afford to pay for medical services continued to do so. By 1916 the Rural Municipalities Act had been amended to allow municipalities to guarantee their physician an annual retainer of $1,500. By 1919 the farm economy had weakened as the price of wheat dropped to a low of $2.63 per bushel, and legislation now allowed individual jurisdictions to guarantee a physician's income up to $5,000 a year.[5] Any municipality could thus employ a physician to provide medical care for all its residents.

The co-operation and solidarity necessary in such situations were rooted in the socioeconomic conditions of the province. Co-operation allowed farmers to pool their resources and continue farming, even though their incomes were low. On the economic level, co-operation soon developed into political action. The Saskatchewan Wheat Pool, the Saskatchewan Co-operative Livestock Marketing Association, the Saskatchewan Co-operative Poultry Producers Limited, and the Saskatchewan Co-operative Creameries were all organized by 1924. In 1930 the United Farmers of Canada, Saskatchewan Section, realizing that urban politicians were more interested in industrialization than in the price of wheat, formed the Farmers' Political Association, contesting a federal election on a platform that included a proposal for state-funded medical care.[6] The extent of their popular support was evident in the fact that they received 23% of the vote in the ridings they contested.

By 1921 the urban population of Saskatchewan had grown to 128,000.[7] Cities became trade centres, providing supplies and services which could not be obtained in rural areas. Packing houses, cold storage plants, an automobile assembly plant, a flour mill, and a CPR hotel were all constructed to encourage industrialization in various cities.

In December 1930 the price of wheat plummeted to 50¢ a bushel on the Winnipeg market. The average per capita income in Saskatchewan fell from $478 in 1929 to $135 in 1933.[8] Municipalities, unable to raise adequate revenues to pay their doctors, sought help from the newly established Saskatchewan Relief Commission and from the Conservative government.

The government responded in November 1931 with a medical relief scheme to help maintain doctors' incomes. Under the plan, physicians in severe drought areas would receive $75 a month, while those in more favourable circumstances would receive $40 a month. In the summer of 1932 the scheme was amended to give relief only to those doctors who were practising in the main drought areas. From November 1933, doctors in severe drought areas received $75 a month and all others received $35.

These schemes did not absolve municipalities of their responsibility for paying doctors' fees and salaries; they merely maintained physicians' incomes so that they would continue practising. Doctors accepted the money because it was often their only source of guaranteed income. Indeed, the relief schemes sheltered the medical profession and allowed physicians to maintain above-average incomes throughout the Depression. A doctor receiving $75 a month under the 1933 relief scheme, for example, would enjoy an annual income of at least $900 at a time when the average per capita income was $135.[a]

The relief schemes may have helped some municipalities to keep their doctors, but they did little to improve the distribution of physicians in the province, and nothing at all to improve economic conditions for other people. Many rural areas continued to go without adequate medical services.

In 1932 the United Farmers of Canada, Saskatchewan Section, joined with the Independent Labour Party to form the Farmers' Labour Party (FLP). Their objectives were embodied in a 15-point program which included public credit, publicly owned resources and utilities, protection from farm and home foreclosure, education reform,

[a] On the municipal doctor (and hospital) schemes, see C. Stuart Houston, *Steps on the Road to Medicare: Why Saskatchewan Led the Way* (Montreal: McGill-Queen's University Press, 2002), chapter 3, and Joan Feather and Vincent L. Matthews, "Early Medical Care in Saskatchewan," *Saskatchewan History* 37, no. 2 (1984): 41–54.

workers' rights, social security, and socialized health care.[9] The Urban Municipalities Association supported the FLP, and in 1933 resolved that "the provincial government immediately institute a plan for state medical and hospital services."[10] Health care became an important political issue for farmers, labourers, politicians, and the medical profession.

Most rural physicians, separated from one another by long distances, were poorly organized. Urban doctors, on the other hand, were able to lobby effectively for their own interests, which did not always coincide with the interests of their rural colleagues. Many rural doctors, for example, were accepting salaries for their services, whereas urban physicians were not. The latter feared that salaried service would limit the possibilities for increasing the incomes they enjoyed under the existing structure of urban medicine. They therefore organized to protect their right to bill patients on a fee-for-service basis, and in 1933 the Saskatchewan Medical Association endorsed private health insurance as the only acceptable means of providing health care.[11] Such insurance allowed urban physicians to set their own fees for services to relief patients. By 1934 the government was providing funds for poor patients on a fee-for-service basis to physicians in Regina, Saskatoon, and Prince Albert.[12]

In 1935, complaining that many municipalities had defaulted on salary payments to rural doctors, their urban colleagues began lobbying the newly elected Liberals to expand the fee-for-service principle to rural municipalities. But the Liberals feared that giving in to the doctors' demands would only increase the popularity of the newly formed Co-operative Commonwealth Federation (CCF), which had developed partly out of the FLP and had adopted much of its platform. The Liberals therefore increased relief grants to doctors in the severe drought areas to $100 per month.[13]

Various organizations continued to campaign for changes in health care services. In 1936 the State Hospital and Medical League was formed to educate and lobby for socialized health care. Over several years it attracted the support of a wide range of governmental and voluntary organizations, including the Saskatchewan Teachers' Federation, the United Farmers of Canada, the Wheat Pool, farm women's organizations, and both rural and urban municipal associations.[14]

The Liberals, however, were opposed to the concept; they believed that socialized health care would interfere with capital development in the province. Instead they proposed that individual citizens be held responsible for paying for their medical services, an ideology that won the support of business and professional groups. The first step in their strategy was to take control of relief grants for medical care. Accordingly, in 1937 they centralized administration of the payments in one provincial agency, the Relief Medical Services Plan.

The medical profession supported the plan because it adopted the existing fee schedule set by physicians in urban centres. Thus, urban physicians were paid on a fee-for-service basis for the care of indigent patients, and they could still bill other patients privately. The incomes of rural physicians also improved as the Liberals increased their relief grants to $250 a month.[15]

But again, provincial relief schemes did not improve accessibility to medical care for people in rural areas. Many municipalities in severe drought areas began to recruit doctors from other countries. The medical profession responded by refusing to grant them licenses to practice. They feared that recruiting foreign doctors for salaried service

The Health Services REVIEW

PUBLISHED IN THE INTERESTS OF ADEQUATE MEDICAL AND HOSPITAL CARE REGARDLESS OF THE ABILITY OF THE INDIVIDUAL TO PAY

Vol. II Regina, Saskatchewan, May, 1946 No. 1

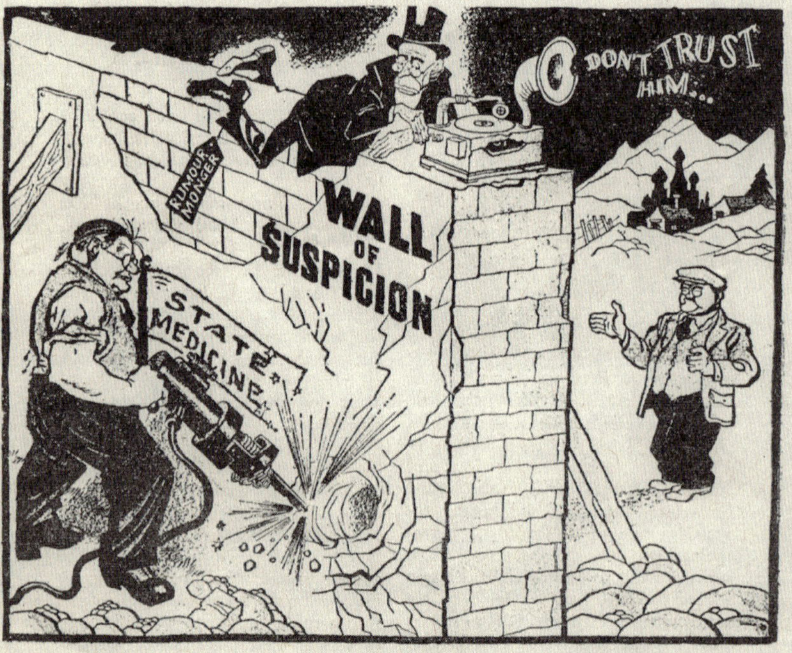

The death struggle of any deep-rooted system is always marked by evidences of suspicion, prejudice and gross misconceptions.

THIS IS HAPPENING IN CANADA

"The 'Wall of Suspicion' towards state medicine," State Hospital and Medical League, *Health Services Review* 11, no. 1 (Regina, May 1946) (SAB Pamphlet Collection G87.1, State Hospital and Medical League).

would lead to an expansion of salaried service throughout the province. They also knew that adding to the medical population could potentially reduce the incomes of doctors already practising. Thus, licensed physicians refused to service drought-stricken areas, while doctors who were willing to do so were unable to obtain licenses.

From 1909 onward, successive provincial governments had supported the medical profession with legislation, protective policies, and subsidies. At no time did doctors suffer financially. The Liberals carried on the tradition. Soon after the election of 1938 they began promoting voluntary health insurance plans as an alternative to universal prepaid health care. The Saskatchewan Mutual Medical and Hospital Benefit Association Act, passed in 1938, enabled any 10 or more persons to incorporate a health insurance plan, provided that an annual report and a financial statement be submitted to an official of the Department of Public Health, and that by-laws, rules, regulations, assessment fees, benefits, and all amendments be subject to the approval of the Department of Health.[16] The first voluntary health insurance plans were established in 1939.

Early plans fell into two distinct categories: consumer sponsored and doctor sponsored. The Regina Rural Medical Benefit Association was a co-operative headed by H.L. Fowler, manager of Consumers' Co-operative Refineries Limited. The co-operative collected 80¢ a month from its membership, and provided medical services in return. They attempted to hire doctors on a salary of $7,200 a year, but the provincial Medical Association disapproved, claiming that the proposed salary was too low to provide adequate service; they also feared that control of medical services would fall into the hands of people who weren't doctors. As a result, the co-operative was forced to reorganize on a fee-for-service basis. The Saskatoon Mutual Medical and Hospital Association, a consumer co-operative modelled after the Regina plan, was organized in the same year, 1939. The Regina District Medical Society organized its own health insurance plan, Medical Services Incorporated (MSI), also in 1939. The plan was incorporated under the Companies Act, and therefore did not have to supply any details of its by-laws, rules and regulations, assessment fees, or benefits to the Department of Health. In later years, the doctor-sponsored plans became dominant, and the co-operatives were forced either to merge with them or be rendered weak alternatives.

Many rural municipalities, hard hit by the drought, hadn't the resources to cover the costs of voluntary health insurance plans. Once again, they took the initiative. In 1939 the rural area of McKillop, without legislative authority, introduced a universal contributory health insurance plan, collecting premiums through taxation from all residents to provide medical care. To accommodate the plan, and others like it, the provincial government passed the Municipal Medical and Hospital Services Act in 1939, permitting municipalities to levy a personal tax or a property tax, or a combination of the two, on each resident of the municipality, provided the personal tax did not exceed $50 a year per family. Universal contributions allowed municipalities to distribute the costs of health care so that all residents were insured for medical services.

Even so, the burden on municipalities during the Depression was intolerable. From 1930 to 1937 Saskatchewan had the highest relief costs in Canada.[17] Total relief expenditures during the period amounted to nearly two-thirds of municipal-provincial revenues. The federal government began formulating policies which would transfer income from wealthier regions to poorer ones. The resultant grant-in-aid policy provided $162 per capita to Saskatchewan for relief purposes, but a major consequence of federal aid was that the province lost its financial independence; during these years, 85% of total relief expenditures came from Dominion loans.

The Royal Commission on Dominion-Provincial Relations was appointed in 1937 by Prime Minister Mackenzie King. King recognized that Saskatchewan and Manitoba were in financial straits and could not continue to provide needed public services. The situation had led to unrest among the unemployed, the working poor, and farmers. King recognized that this unrest was strengthening the popularity of the CCF. The commission was therefore instructed to examine the economic basis of the distribution of legislative power.[18] In particular, it was to investigate the character and the amount of taxes collected and to determine whether taxation was both equitable and efficient. King also instructed the commission to examine the constitutional allocation of revenue sources and determine the relationship of federal and provincial control over these resources. In 1940 the commission released its recommendations in the Rowell-Sirois Report.

The Rowell-Sirois Report made history during the war years. The federal government, with control of military production and monetary and fiscal policies, was able unilaterally to implement the recommendations proposed in it. The report advocated that personal and corporate income tax be under the control of the federal government, and that the provinces keep the lesser social services while the Dominion assume unemployment insurance, contributory old age pensions, jurisdiction over minimum wages, maximum hours, and minimum age of employment. Ottawa was also to assume provincial debts and provide the provinces with National Adjustment Grants based on their fiscal needs.

The Rowell-Sirois Report also recommended that Ottawa supervise all insurance companies, except those that were confined to one province. This meant that the voluntary plans set up by the medical profession in Saskatchewan were accountable to neither the provincial nor the federal government. Under the Companies Act, they were free to set premium rates, determine eligibility for benefits, and control fee schedules. Subscribers to the doctor-controlled plans had no voice in the way the plans were administered, and there was no procedure for electing non-medical members to their boards of directors.[b]

In 1944, the first CCF government was elected to the provincial legislature on a platform that included a complete system of socialized health services. Premier T.C. Douglas, who was also Minister of Health, appointed Dr. Henry E. Sigerist[c] to head a Health Services Study Commission for the purpose of studying existing services and proposing ways to extend them. The commission met across Saskatchewan and considered briefs from about 100 groups and individuals.

In October 1944 Sigerist submitted his report to the government.[19] He recommended the establishment of a Health Services Planning Commission to implement

[b] The Saskatchewan government's negotiating positions on health insurance during the Rowell-Sirois Commission and the subsequent Dominion-Provincial Reconstruction Conference is set out by Joan Feather in "Horse-Trading and Health Insurance: Saskatchewan and Dominion-Provincial Relations, 1937–1947," *Saskatchewan History* 39, no. 3 (1986): 94–106.

[c] Jacalyn Duffin, "The Guru and the Godfather: Henry Sigerist, Hugh MacLean, and the Politics of Health Reform in 1940s Canada," *Canadian Bulletin of Medical History* 9 (1992): 191–218. Jacalyn Duffin and Leslie A. Falk, "Sigerist in Saskatchewan: The Quest for Balance in Social and Technical Medicine," *Bulletin of the History of Medicine* 70, no. 2 (1996): 658–83.

health programs in the province. He also suggested that the province be divided into health districts, each having a District Health Centre headed by a full-time Medical Officer of Health. Sigerist believed that "such decentralization of activities would increase the efficiency of the public health and medical services, while the principle of centralized direction will be maintained."[20] A district hospital, he said, should be located near the Health Centre and employ at least one full-time surgeon. He further recommended that rural municipalities organize into health units to be comprised of one or more municipalities and the towns and villages located therein. Each rural health unit would have its Health Services Commission, with broad representation from the communities involved. Representatives of the local Health Services Commissions and of the District Hospitals would constitute the District Health Services Commission which the District Health Officer would head. Under such a system, Sigerist wrote:

> ...the member of a farm family who becomes sick will seek advice at the Rural Health Centre, or will be visited at home by the municipal doctor. At the Rural Health Centre patients requiring specialized treatment or surgery would be referred to the large centres in Saskatoon, Moose Jaw, or Regina.[21]

Sigerist also recommended the expansion of training programs for nurses, physiotherapists, social workers, and dentists. He found that, although accessibility to health care was not an urgent problem in urban areas, there were city-dwellers who could not afford the premiums of the voluntary insurance plans. He thus recommended a scheme of compulsory insurance in the cities, and further recommended that free hospitalization be available to all residents of the province, and that all medical personnel be put on salary:

> The number of practicing physicians in the province is far too small to give adequate service to the entire population. The only remedies to increase the number of physicians is to make conditions of practice more attractive. Salaries paid at present are too low and the salary scale should be revised and graded according to experience and responsibility. The Medical School of the University will be upgraded so as to train physicians of social medical service.[22]

In November 1944 the CCF appointed the Health Services Planning Commission according to the recommendations made by Dr. Sigerist, and the work of the Commission followed the guidelines laid down in his report. The Commission completed its work in February 1945, and reported its findings to the Department of Health. Its proposals included the regional organization of medical services, compulsory health insurance, and centralized planning and administration:

Many aspects of health service require intimate interest and participation of the people concerned, and this can best be obtained if they have a measure of responsibility and control. In Saskatchewan there is a long tradition of local initiative and self-help. In many areas municipalities provide residents with a close approach to ideal services that can at present be provided on a provincial scale. The way must be left open for them to continue to do this. It will therefore be necessary to plan a combination of centralized planning and supervision, plus financial assistance, with considerable responsibility left in the hands of the local bodies. Until a province wide financial basis can be arranged an equalization grant will have to be paid by the provincial Government, in addition to a subsidy for all units adopting the model plan.[23]

The Health Services Planning Commission recommended that the province provide assistance for building health centres, but that their maintenance should be a local responsibility, aided by grants. It further advised that general practitioners should be paid by salary, as this had proven to be a satisfactory method of providing medical care in small centres and rural areas. The Commission also believed that it would encourage the doctor to concentrate more on preventative work, since studies had shown that municipal doctors on salary did more such work than those who were paid on a fee-for-service basis. It removed the temptation to do unnecessary work, or work for which a particular doctor might not be qualified. It also allowed doctors to budget for the cost of such service and to plan retirement, paid holiday time, post-graduate work, and so on. Under the suggested contract, the doctor would be Medical Officer of Health unless a region was established with full-time public health workers. Doctors would be supplied with rent-free quarters, equipment, instruments, and drugs. They would also have the right to appeal dismissal and to request transfer.[d]

The proposed plan would be financed by grants, but these were not intended to relieve local communities of their responsibilities. Rather, the grants would be of two kinds: a flat sum to maintain the standard of service, and equalization grants for poorer communities that were having trouble financing health care services.

The medical profession did not approve. MSI had always been free under the Companies Act to enter into agreements with municipalities virtually without restriction on premiums, benefits, and fee schedules. The company encouraged municipalities to join its plan, and doctors favoured MSI because it offered fee-for-service payment. To create a successful regional health service, the CCF had to obstruct these contracts. The Health Services Act therefore consolidated all legislative provisions authorizing health service insurance programs, and prohibited municipalities from entering into contracts with doctor-controlled plans. The Companies Act, however, was still without restriction in terms of the contracts it could procure. The laws were contradictory, ineffective, and not enforced.

In 1946 the Swift Current Health Region was established as a pilot program.[e] Basic health services were to be organized, with the costs shared by the province and the region. All residents of the region of 90 days' standing were eligible for services, with no penalty imposed for non-payment of the tax. The municipality was held responsible for the payment of unpaid personal tax at the end of each year. The plan included the use of utilization fees for office and home calls.

One year after the Swift Current Health Region had opened its medical care program, the CCF established the Saskatchewan Hospital Services Plan. Although the program was working well in Swift Current, the government was unable to extend it

[d] See Gordon S. Lawson, "The Road Not Taken: The 1945 Health Services Planning Commission Proposals and Physician Remuneration in Saskatchewan," *Canadian Bulletin of Medical History* 26, no. 2 (2009): 395–427.

[e] See Joan Feather's two articles on the early introduction of universal hospital and medical care insurance in this health region: "From Concept to Reality: Formation of the Swift Current Health Region," *Prairie Forum* 16, no. 1 (1991): 59–80; and "Impact of the Swift Current Health Region: Experiment of Model?" *Prairie Forum* 16, no. 2 (1991): 225–48.

province-wide because of lack of funding. Premier Douglas proposed to undertake a comprehensive program of medical care when the federal government began paying a share of the costs of the existing plan. Until this occurred, people who could afford to insure themselves against the costs of medical care had to do so through the voluntary plans. Between 1944 and 1954, however, 84 hospitals were built in rural areas, with the province offering grants to municipalities for equipment and staff.

The medical profession, opposed to any reduction of its control over medical practice, promoted the expansion of voluntary health insurance plans. Medical Services Incorporated (MSI) and Group Medical Services (GMS) began a campaign to encourage their philosophy. MSI wanted to insure residents of municipalities on a per capita rate for a fixed period. The Minister of Health advised municipalities that they did not have the authority to enter into such agreements. Municipalities, nevertheless, were forced to enter into contracts with MSI when their doctors terminated their municipal agreements:

> Municipalities felt that their residents wanted medical care insurance to continue and when local doctors would not continue with the local agreements there was no alternative to the contract offered by MSI... The municipalities did not fear the consequences of legal action or legislative reprisal because there was none.[24]

MSI lobbied the government to amend the Health Services Act so that municipalities could allow corporations to enter into agreements with their residents. MSI further wanted the government to lift the $50 personal tax maximum so that plans would not be dependent on municipal revenues. The CCF refused, believing that the municipality should retain administrative and financial control of its health care program. If corporations became insurers, they could set per capita premiums, leading to private profit. The government also refused to increase the personal tax levy because more than $50 a year would be prohibitive for many families in many communities. The Department of Health advised municipalities not to exceed statutory authority, but took no formal action against those which did.

Consumer-sponsored health plans languished, accumulated deficits, and either died or were swallowed by larger corporations. In contrast, MSI and GMS flourished. In 1958, MSI held subscriptions with 22% of the population. GMS entered into group contracts with employment and commercial organizations, and in 1950 had the largest voluntary plan in the province.[f]

The voluntary health insurance plans were costly to operate. Premiums were out of reach of many people, and the chronically ill were often excluded because they were bad risks. Nevertheless, voluntary plans were strongly supported by the medical profession. With such plans in place, doctors could control their conditions of work and mode of payment. The CCF did little to oppose them: it was politically dangerous when physicians could terminate contracts and leave people without health care. Besides, the plans reduced government health care expenses. The CCF concentrated instead on establishing health regions and providing hospital care.

[f] On the significance of the physician-sponsored insurance plans in struggle against universal medical care insurance by organized medicine in Canada (and the United States), see C. David Naylor, *Private Practice, Public Payment: Canadian Medicine and the Politics of Health Insurance, 1911–1966* (Montreal: McGill-Queen's University Press, 1986).

Notes

1. A. Artibise, *Prairie Urban Development 1870–1930* (Booklet 34, 1981), 31.

2. Interdepartmental Committee to Study Medical Care Insurance, "Organized Medicine's Official Position on Health Insurance" (1959), 1.

3. *Royal Commission on Medical Manpower in Canada* (Ottawa: Queen's Printer, 1964).

4. R.F. Badgley and S. Wolfe, "Medical Care and Conflict in Saskatchewan," *Milbank Memorial Fund Quarterly* 43, nos. 463–79 (1967): 72.

5. Interdepartmental Committee Report, 1959.

6. John F. Conway, *The West* (Toronto: James Lorimer and Company, 1984), bibliography.

7. Artibise, *Prairie Urban Development 1870–1930.*

8. Conway, *The West*, 104.

9. Ibid., 133.

10. M.G. Taylor, *Health Insurance and Canadian Public Policy* (Montreal: Queen's University Press, 1978), 74.

11. Ibid., 241.

12. Saskatchewan Medical Association, "Provision for medical care of relief recipients in the cities of Saskatchewan," *Saskatchewan Medical Quarterly* 2, no. 1 (1938): 12.

13. Saskatchewan Medical Association, "Assistance to Municipalities Re: Provision of Medical Dervices in the Dried Out Areas," *Saskatchewan Medical Quarterly* 1, no. 3 (1937): 9.

14. Conway, *The West*.

15. Saskatchewan Department of Public Health, *Annual Report*, 1937.

Interdepartmental Committee Report, 3.

Donald V. Smiley, *The Rowell-Sirois Report, Book 1* (Toronto: The Macmillan Company of Canada Ltd, 1978), 177.

18. Ibid., 3.

19. Health Services Survey Commission, Report of the Commissioner Henry E. Sigerist, MD, Presented to the Minister of Public Health, October 4th (Regina: King's Printer, 1947).

20. Ibid., 4.

21. Ibid., 6.

22. Ibid., 10.

23. Department of Public Health, Health Services Planning Commission, "Report on Regional Health Services—A Proposed Plan" (1945), 3.

24. Interdepartmental Committee to Study Medical Care Insurance, "Voluntary Medical Care Plans in Saskatchewan" (1958).

Chapter 2
A Brief History of Organized Medicine

Before 1860, medicine was not recognized as a profession in Canada. Doctors constituted a minority among practitioners of the healing arts. On the prairies especially, people would often use a local healer rather than travel long distances to obtain a physician's care. Doctors were more plentiful in Eastern Canada, especially in the urban areas where immigrant physicians from the United States and England had settled. When the first medical school was established in 1850, the movement to professionalize medicine, and thus gain control of the health care system across Canada, was begun.[1]

As the success of herbalists and midwives and the like reduced the credibility of physicians, a key step in the professionalization of medicine was to exclude alternate healers from the realm of medical care. To accomplish this, physicians had to control licensing, and to control licensing they had to organize. In 1869 the College of Physicians and Surgeons of Ontario was established, and soon gained control over the licensing of all healing practitioners in Ontario. Non-medical healing practices thus came under the jurisdiction of organized medicine.

Although the College had the right to control licensing in Ontario, it could do little to regulate medical practice in other provinces. Physicians feared that public acceptance of alternate healers in the rest of Canada would threaten the autonomy of the medical profession in Ontario. This concern was partially addressed by the Medical Practitioners Ordinance, passed in 1885, which required doctors across Canada to register their practices. But whereas the Act provided Ontario physicians with information about who was practising medicine, it did not allow them to enforce licensing regulations. By the next decade, however, the College had gained control of licensing procedures across Canada.

In the United States, doctors had organized in 1847, establishing the American Medical Association. Physicians were plentiful at the time; anyone with a medical diploma could practise medicine, and diplomas were readily obtainable through commercial schools, or even by mail. Aside from quite valid concerns about the competence of such practitioners, their general availability threatened the livelihood of more orthodox physicians. An explicit purpose of the AMA, therefore, was to exclude diploma doctors from the practice of medicine. They accepted funding from American corporations to finance their campaign.[a]

[a] This change is described in great detail by Paul Starr, *The Social Transformation of American Medicine: The Rise of a Sovereign Profession and the Making of a Vast Industry* (New York: Basic Books, 1984).

In 1909 the Carnegie Foundation supported a proposal from the AMA to review medical education.[2] Abraham Flexner, appointed by the Foundation, proceeded to evaluate the quality of medical schools in both the United States and Canada. He criticized most of them for their failure to enforce preliminary education requirements, their inadequate facilities, insufficient training in laboratory sciences and clinical medicine, and for their over-production of doctors. Flexner recommended that medical education be based on a uniform scientific doctrine: the germ theory of disease. To facilitate this, he proposed that medical schools be affiliated with universities. Corporations used the Flexner report to downplay the need for costly workplace and public health reforms—the cause of worker illness and death, after all, had been shown to be faulty medical practice, not a poisonous environment—and the AMA used the report to close the diploma medical schools.

Flexner's report changed the face of medical education. Based on the germ theory of disease, it became cure-oriented rather than preventative.[3] Medical practice moved from the application of practical skills toward an increasing dependence on technology. Flexner thus helped not only to professionalize medical practice, but at the same time encouraged the development of corporate medical supply industries.[b]

The move to "scientize" medicine across Canada began in Ontario, where the growth of industry was more widespread than in any other province.[4] Industrialization was necessarily accompanied by rapid urbanization and its attendant problems among the working class and the poor. In 1909, on the advice of the American scientific management expert Gifford Pinchot, the federal Liberals established a Commission on Conservation. The Commission found that the lack of adequate housing, nutritious food, and proper sanitation in urban areas was creating a high death rate from communicable diseases and poverty-related illnesses. In 1910, for example, the death rate from communicable diseases in Toronto was 114 per 100,000 population.[5] The Commission instituted public health programs—including sewage treatment, nursing services, and the distribution of fresh milk among the poor—and by 1914 managed to reduce the death rate to 27 per 100,000.

Under the leadership of Wilfrid Laurier, the Liberals implemented public health reforms, hoping to build support among the working class. It cost them support in the corporate sector and in the medical profession, however, for the success of the programs demonstrated that medical treatment was not the only means of improving the health of the electorate, and this knowledge threatened the livelihood of Ontario physicians. Public health reforms were also costly to corporate profits, and, shortly after the reforms were implemented, doctors and industrialists in Ontario joined forces to protect their interests and to ensure that the Liberals were not re-elected.[6]

In 1911 the Rockefeller Foundation began to support the germ theory approach to medical education. It offered endowments to medical schools in the United States and in Canada, conditional on the establishment of full-time clinical professorships. By 1921, the Foundation had spent some $45 million on medical education.[7] The schools were dependent on endowments to upgrade their facilities and to keep their accreditation, and responsibility for health was effectively shifted from industry to medical science.

[b] On Flexner's impact, see Thomas Neville Bonner, *Iconoclast: Abraham Flexner and a Life in Learning* (Baltimore: Johns Hopkins University Press, 2002).

Ontario physicians knew that widespread public health measures would lower the prestige of "scientific" medicine, so in 1911 the College of Physicians and Surgeons of Ontario established the Canadian Medical Association. One of the Association's founding fathers was Sir Charles Tupper, a Conservative politician who had been defeated by Laurier in the general election of 1900. Tupper and his colleagues supported the Ontario physicians in their campaign to defeat the Liberals in the upcoming general election.

Conservative political support was vital to the CMA's bid to control medical practice across the country. Initially, the CMA focused on building its membership. Of the 7,000 doctors practising in Canada in 1911, only 1,400 were members of the CMA, and the bulk of them were from the east. The first step, therefore, was to encourage physicians in the Western provinces to join the Association. The *Montreal Medical Journal* and the *Maritime Medical News* were amalgamated in 1911 to become the official CMA *Journal*, which was used to educate and inform the membership of the policies adopted by the CMA.[8] One year after the defeat of the Laurier government, the Conservatives passed the Canada Medical Act (1912) which gave the CMA the power to control licensing procedures for medical practice across Canada.

During the war years the CMA was weak and relatively inactive, as many Ontario physicians were serving overseas. The Association continued to be national in name only; by 1914 only the Maritimes, Manitoba, and Alberta had joined Ontario in the CMA.[9] An executive was elected at the annual meeting in St John's in 1914, but no further meetings were held until after World War I.

The American Medical Association, meanwhile, had become stronger. Legislatures had granted it the right to determine accreditation standards for hospitals, and for the training of nurses and technicians. It had succeeded in outlawing non-medical healing practices, which were labelled "unscientific" and "quackery."[10] By 1914, the dominance of the medical profession was unchallenged in the American health system.

In Canada at this time, public health programs were based on precedents set by voluntary relief agencies, with little input from the medical profession. Ontario physicians criticized the CMA's inability to control provincial medical associations; they objected when physicians in rural Saskatchewan, for example, agreed to work for a salary when the Rural Municipalities Act (1916) was passed. They criticized the CMA for its lack of political action in the face of federal legislation that would impinge on professional autonomy. The AMA had clearly demonstrated that an organized profession would be powerful enough to protect its own interests and to affect the outcome of health policies. This was the security coveted by Ontario physicians, and if the CMA were to gain control of medical practice it would have to reorganize.

At the 1919 annual meeting of the CMA, a resolution was passed calling for revision of the Association's constitution and by-laws. A committee was appointed to work toward the incorporation of all provincial medical associations under the CMA constitution. Provincial associations resisted, however, and in 1920 a new resolution was put forward at the annual meeting: that provincial associations become branches of the CMA while maintaining their own constitutions and by-laws. Following the meeting, Ontario physicians disaffiliated themselves from the CMA.

At the Ontario Medical Association's annual meeting in 1920, the membership decided to publish its own journal, and subsequently contracted with Macmillan Publishing to produce the *Canadian Medical Monthly*, the official journal of the Association.[11] The OMA controlled all copy, text, and advertising under the direction of an editorial board appointed by the OMA.

In the same year the Executive Council of the Canadian Medical Association—at that time an organization with less than 1,000 members and debts totalling $14,000—approached the OMA with a view to editorial collaboration, for without the Ontario physicians' support, the CMA was essentially powerless. Macmillan subsequently sold the *Canadian Medical Monthly* to the CMA for $1,200 and, by 1921, the CMA *Journal* was under the control of the Ontario Medical Association. Hence, the interests of Ontario physicians, who were urban based and of largely British and American backgrounds, became the interests of Canadian medicine as a whole.

The nucleus of the CMA was comprised of doctors from urban Ontario. They knew that if they did not gain control over provincial associations, physicians outside Ontario would accept working conditions contrary to the interest of urban practice. At the 1921 annual meeting of the CMA, a plan of reorganization was approved. The plan provided for a full-time position of Secretary, who was responsible for the advancement of the organization on a national scale. The plan also provided that the CMA would be the governing body for all provincial medical associations.

By 1929, health insurance had become a major concern of the CMA, as it recognized that depressed economies in the Western provinces made state involvement in medical care attractive. A Committee on Economics was appointed to study the issue and formulate a coherent statement for the Association. In 1934 the CMA released its Plan for Health Insurance in Canada. The Association contended that the state should provide funding for medical services for indigent persons, but that people who could afford it should be responsible for their own health insurance. Not surprisingly, the health insurance plans endorsed by the CMA were voluntary and private.

The Ontario physicians established a Medical Welfare Plan, which they controlled, in 1935. Funding from the Ontario government was used to remunerate the OMA for the medical care of some 350,000 relief recipients. This was the first time in Canada that funds for the health insurance of a substantial proportion of the population were turned over to a voluntary medical body for administration and distribution. Within two years, the Ontario physicians had established their own voluntary health insurance plans, the Associated Medical Services Plan and the Windsor Medical Services Plan.[12] These plans were supported by the profession, and by 1939 the entire provincial association had come under the control of the CMA.

The CMA used its *Journal* to control the profession ideologically, to communicate its ideas and policies to physicians across Canada. The advertising for pharmaceuticals, the articles on new research and current affairs, all contributed to the values that practising physicians held in regard to their own medical practice. The *Journal* associated technology and specialization with superiority, CMA policies with self-determination.

The emphasis on self-determination was not unique to the CMA. In 1920, the American Medical Association, fearing that public financing would lead to public control of medical practice, had opposed health insurance regulation by any state or federal government. The AMA saw health insurance as a threat to its independence and, like the CMA, proposed that health insurance be carried through private companies.

The first hospitalization insurance emerged out of a 1929 arrangement between the school teachers of Dallas, Texas, and Baylor University Hospital. The hospital proposed that teachers, who were otherwise unable to pay their individual hospital bills, pay the hospital a monthly fee. In return, the hospital guaranteed each teacher up to 21 days' use of a semi-private room and other hospital services at no further charge. This first "Blue Cross" plan had two characteristics which became the pattern for other such plans: it provided service benefits, and it was controlled by the hospital. By 1933, Blue Cross plans had been established in California and New Jersey. State legislatures supported the plans by making them tax exempt and by not interfering with their operation. By 1940, Blue Cross had six million subscribers in the United States.[13]

Blue Cross is owned by the American Hospital Association, and subscribers have no say in how the plan is managed. The typical plan provides for a self-recruited board of trustees, with doctors holding one-third of the seats, hospital administrators another third, and alternate representatives the last third. The latter are appointed by the hospital-medical establishment and are mostly business people.[14] When hospitals negotiate contracts with Blue Cross, they are in effect negotiating with themselves.[c]

The growth of hospital insurance plans incidentally increased the medical profession's dependence on technology. The plans made hospitals economically viable and provided capital for new equipment, which in turn created a dependence on diagnostic and treatment technology which was only available in hospitals. Doctors could no longer stock their offices with the equipment necessary to diagnose and treat disease, because it was too expensive. Inevitably, the medical profession's dependence on technology increased the profits of corporations involved in the manufacture of medical equipment.

American physicians feared that hospital insurance would lead to medical insurance—not unreasonably, in view of the easy acceptance of hospital insurance by state legislatures and the public. In 1934, the AMA proposed that all features of medical service should be under the control of the medical profession, and that no third party be permitted to enter the patient-physician relationship.[15] It was also in 1934, however, that Franklin Roosevelt decided to act more aggressively in the matter of social welfare reform, establishing a Committee on Economic Security to "study problems related to the economic security of individuals."[16] Relatively early in the Committee's deliberation, it became clear that the administration was having difficulties including compulsory health insurance in its proposals. Not surprisingly, the AMA was involved.

In 1934, the Association passed a program known as the "AMA Ten Principles" which set out guidelines for medical societies in regard to the implementation of health insurance. The AMA, followed by the CMA, demanded that any medical service plan be under the control of the medical profession, and that the medical profession be solely responsible for the character of the service provided. It insisted on doctors' rights to choose patients. It also insisted that the cost of medical services be paid by the patient.

Public demand for the extension of medical services and the relief of medical costs was persistent, however, and led to a National Health Conference in Washington in

[c] For a history of Blue Cross, see Robert Cunningham III and Robert M. Cunningham Jr., *The Blues: A History of the Blue Cross and Blue Shield Systems* (DeKalb: Northern Illinois University Press, 1997). For its influence in Canada, see Terry Boychuk, *The Making and Meaning of Hospital Policy in the United States and Canada* (Ann Arbor: University of Michigan Press, 1999), 91–92, 109–11.

1938. At the conference, the AMA warned against federal intervention in medical economics because it could lower the quality of treatment. Nevertheless, the conference adopted a National Health Program which called for federal assistance in the construction of hospitals and health clinics, the expansion of public health services, and improved accessibility to medical care through compulsory insurance and taxation.

In 1939, the Wagner Bill was introduced federally, calling for $35 million in federal grants to the states to finance health care. A National Committee for the Extension of Medical Services was formed to kill it. The Committee was established as an independent organization but its relationship with the AMA was obvious and intimate. Its activities included public awareness campaigns, educating physicians and their patients about government health insurance, and lobbying the government. The Committee's treasury was aided principally by contributions from the pharmaceutical industry. By 1943 the Wagner Bill had died.

On other fronts, an encouraging public response to the costs of medical care was the Group Health Association which insured government employees. The AMA campaigned to obstruct the GHA's attempts to hire qualified doctors or use existing medical and hospital facilities. The GHA responded with an antitrust conspiracy suit against the AMA, which it won in 1939, thus opening the door for co-operative plans across the United States.[17]

The Farm Security Administration was an important force in educating the public to the advantages of federal participation in medical care.[18] The FSA provided the stimulus for co-operative plans, under which members paid an annual fee to the co-operative and, in turn, were guaranteed medical services for the current year. As the drought had hit the mid-west states in 1936–37, the majority of farm families were unable to afford medical care, and many rural doctors were unable to collect fees for services provided. In the face of this crisis, the program of rural co-operatives mushroomed, and eventually covered 88 counties in 43 states. In the peak year, 1943, half a million persons were covered by co-operatives.[d]

During the 1930s, several medical societies organized voluntary insurance plans which transferred the responsibility of collecting fees from the individual practitioner to the local medical society. The plans fell into two categories: those which permitted low-income patients to budget for their individual medical bills after they were incurred, and those that catered to the middle class and incorporated group repayment.

Medical indemnity plans were also developed during the Depression. These featured pre-payment, choice of doctor, and broad coverage, and met most of the needs of the middle class. Patients paid an annual fee, but had little control over the administration

[d] Currently, there are three large health maintenance organizations in the United States incorporated as consumer co-operatives providing services to approximately two million individuals. The co-operative form is also present in other health care sectors; however, the goal of these co-operatives in many cases is to benefit the provider of services (such as through joint purchasing), rather than to democratize the provision of health care services, as was Rands's major interest. For a full picture of co-operatives involved in health care delivery in the U.S., see Steve Deller, Ann Hoyt, Brent Hueth and Reka Sundaram-Stukel, *Research on the Economic Impact of Co-operatives* (Madison: University of Wisconsin Center for Co-operatives, 2009). Note that the United States also features a large network of consumer-driven community health centres: see Shelly Raymer Duncan and Cinthia Deye, "Community Health Centers as Primary Providers of Health Care," *Ageing International* 31, no. 2 (2006): 154–67.

of the plan. Physicians remained in private practice and used the plans to guarantee that they would be paid a high percentage of patients' insurance fees. Because the administration lacked control over doctors' fees, these plans were unstable. In the 1940s the number of insured services was reduced, membership fees were increased, and deductible clauses and income ceilings were introduced. The indemnity plans, although unable to service low-income groups, were used as models by state and local plans across the United States and eventually became part of the Blue Shield System.[19]

Group hospitalization plans enjoyed broad support among the middle classes. The American College of Surgeons hoped that this type of insurance would protect patients and hospitals, and maintain the financial position of the middle class membership. Some of the plans received initial funding from philanthropic organizations. Some were controlled by the local medical society and hospital administrators; others were administered by civil leaders and public representatives in co-operation with professional groups. The American Hospital Association made an early attempt to police them, establishing in 1933 a series of guidelines and giving advice to groups interested in founding new plans. The system continued until 1937, when the AHA created the Hospital Service Plan Commission. Financed by the Rosenwald Fund and designed to co-ordinate the plans on a national basis, the Commission created the Blue Cross symbol to signify that a particular plan had met with Hospital Association requirements and was a co-operating member of the national system. From 1934 to 1939, the enrolment and number of hospitalization plans snowballed, and many state governments began to pass legislation permitting the formation of local plans.

The success of voluntary hospitalization plans tended to obscure their shortcomings. Families of members often received only partial coverage; low-income families and independently employed individuals found it hard to join; and medical services, even when used in the hospital, were seldom included in the benefits. During unemployment or following a change of job, a subscriber often lost eligibility for membership, and because they were private businesses, the average subscriber had no input into fees or coverage, not to mention the nature and quality of services provided.

Administrators of the plans were reluctant to include high-risk individuals, low-income families, or farmers. They also avoided paying hospital professional bills, because national and local medical societies had initially opposed group hospitalization as violating the ethical code of the profession and endangering the doctor-patient relationship. Finally, since the bulk of middle class members seemed content with the partial coverage provided by the plans and were not interested in expanding them, there was little momentum to establish consumer controlled, public medical care.

The AMA was the most powerful force opposing further medical care reforms. Its power came from its structure. Every member belonged to a local society. Local societies were federated into state associations which, in turn, were represented on the national level by the AMA. The national leaders were usually conservative, successful doctors who opposed changes in medical practices which might threaten their incomes and control. Most doctors in the 1920s and 1930s trusted the national leadership, believing that high quality medical care was tied to the doctor-patient relationship, free competition, individual initiative, and fee-for-service. These doctors admired the image of the family doctor, frowned on specialization and group practice, and feared and despised any interference in the professional and financial affairs of individual physicians.

When the AMA decided that proposed or existing plans did not conform to their members' ideology or code of ethics, both the Association and its constituent societies took action. They organized political lobbying, propaganda campaigns, and disciplinary actions ranging from the professional ostracism of participating physicians to the intimidation of hospitals and clinics that cooperated against the interests of the AMA.[20]

In the 1930s the Blue Cross and Blue Shield plans competed with the co-operatives for public and professional support. Later, the Farm Security Administration program competed with the Blue plans. Still later, commercial insurance companies presented their own plans. The effect of competition was that each plan had to strive for the most profitable subscribers, the ones with the lowest health risks and the highest degree of acceptance from the providers of the service, the physicians. In the final analysis, it was the medical societies that determined which plans survived and which did not.

In 1948, Harry Truman was elected President of the United States on a platform that included compulsory health insurance. In December of that year the AMA hired a public relations team. Instead of generally denouncing health insurance bills, the AMA promoted the growth of private health insurance plans.[21] By 1949, it had collected almost 2,000 organizational endorsements for voluntary insurance. In 1950, it accelerated the campaign, and the list of endorsements grew to 11,000. Advertisements in the media promoted liberalism and the freedom of the individual to choose voluntary health insurance. Almost 60% of the funding used in the campaign came from business and insurance companies. In 1950, Truman was defeated and Eisenhower elected.[e]

Eisenhower was opposed to compulsory health insurance. He met with the AMA and secured their approval for a Department of Health, Education, and Welfare conditional on the understanding that a position of Special Assistant for Health and Medical Affairs would be created for the medical profession. During Eisenhower's term in office many Social Security services were expanded and health reforms passed.

Then in 1956 the AMA tried to prevent the passage of an amendment to the Social Security Act. Hostility to the law stemmed from a reluctance to grant government the right to determine whether an individual suffered from a medical condition. The AMA also felt that retirement benefits at age 50 might encourage malingering, and by offering cash rewards for infirmity and permanent disabilities the government would encourage individual irresponsibility. The Association contended that the extension of Social Security benefits to the disabled aged 50 or more would lead to complete national health insurance, with coverage for hospitalization, medical treatment, and drugs. The AMA regarded national health insurance as the end to medical freedom.[22]

In 1957, legislation was introduced in the United States whereby individuals eligible for retirement benefits from Social Security would be assured surgical and hospital insurance. With the aid of the American Hospital Association and various insurance companies, the AMA managed to defeat the bill, arguing that medical insurance for the elderly should be held privately. At one point the AMA did call on local medical societies to reduce their fees to the aged, but the financing of health care for the elderly became a major issue in the election of 1960.

[e] This is an error that appeared in the original publication. In fact, there was no election in 1950, but in the 1952 United States election, Adlai Stevenson, the presidential candidate for the Democrats, was defeated by the Republican candidate, Dwight D. Eisenhower. Harry Truman, the outgoing President (a Democrat), did not run for re-election.

It was not until 1965 that Medicare and Medicaid were finally enacted into law. The former was a government-operated insurance program for the elderly. Like conventional insurance, the insured had to pay premiums in the form of payroll taxes. A government subsidy was added to this to bring the total to an amount adequate to insure those over 65. Medicaid worked on different principles. Under Medicaid the government provided matching grants to states and local governments, financed out of general tax revenues, to pay directly for health services used by certain categories of the poor.[23]

In Canada, the CMA followed a parallel course to that of the AMA, against the wishes of many of its own members. By 1929, health insurance was one of the major concerns of the Canadian Medical Association. Brief references to health insurance, mainly commenting on the situation in Great Britain, had appeared in the records of the Association and its *Journal* as early as 1919.[24] The first serious consideration of the matter occurred in 1929, when the Canadian Medical Association's Committee on Economics reported on the Ontario Medical Association's resolution to recommend a government commission to study health insurance and suggest ways of achieving adequate service. Realizing that provincial independence threatened the political power of the CMA, the Committee on Economics set about formulating a national statement.

But the unity of the CMA was fragmented, and several Western provinces had already initiated commissions of inquiry before the CMA had completed its statement. In 1929 and 1933, two Commissions in Alberta had favoured health insurance. In 1933, the medical profession in Saskatchewan endorsed health insurance, and in 1934 the government of British Columbia legislated in favour of health insurance. By 1934, the Committee on Economics recognized that depressed economies in the Western provinces were a real threat to the autonomy of the profession, since physicians in these regions were willing to accept some form of government intervention to protect their incomes. Moreover, the governments themselves were grasping at the prospect of health insurance to strengthen their political positions. The CMA therefore consolidated its policy on health insurance in a report entitled "Plan for Health Insurance in Canada."

The report contained 16 principles on which health insurance should be based. It emphasized the concept of federation, stressing that any plan should recognize the long-term consequences of government action on the profession. But the socioeconomic conditions in the eastern and western regions of Canada were utterly different. Western physicians, having worked in an agrarian society, had learned to accept government involvement in their lives and were committed to co-operative organizations. Eastern physicians worked in a mainly urban, industrialized society and were easily influenced by American policies. Since the bulk of the CMA's membership and leadership was in the east, many of its policies were inappropriate for and insensitive to the needs of western physicians. CMA policies, in fact, became a tool of oppression in terms of any progressive actions western physicians might endorse:

> At the 1940 Annual Convention, the CMA attempted to consolidate its position with the western provinces. "The foundations for a truly medical organization had been well laid. Essential elements guarding provincial autonomy, while making for national cohesion, have been carefully built into the Constitution and By-Laws. It now remains for all the provinces in Canada to build upon this foundation

> a Canadian Medical Association capable of performing all the duties and functions which should devolve upon a medical association."The CMA dictated that the provinces should conform to national policy on any question. At the convention, the General Council was declared the parliament of Canadian medicine. The eastern physicians feared that the western doctors would agree to adopt state-aided health insurance, and this would reduce the profession's power to control the health system.[25]

In 1942 the Government of Canada established the Advisory Committee on Health Insurance, under the chairmanship of Dr. J.J. Heagerty, to plan a measure of health insurance for post-war implementation.[f] A committee of seven was selected by the CMA to work closely with the Committee, which produced a draft bill to provide the model for federal and provincial health insurance plans. The CMA continued to hold meetings during the war years, involving itself in policy decisions on socioeconomic conditions and improving its public image by advocating some social programs. In 1943 the Association declared that the only acceptable health insurance plan was a voluntary health insurance plan.

In 1945 the move toward legislation for health insurance was halted when the Dominion-Provincial Conference on Reconstruction failed to agree on fiscal matters concerning the allocation of funds to the provinces. By 1948 the federal government was ready to implement a compromise on health insurance; after consultation with the CMA, it announced that National Health Grants for hospitals would be offered to the provinces. The government declared that these grants were a fundamental prerequisite to a nation-wide system of health insurance.

The College of Physicians and Surgeons of Saskatchewan, at its annual meeting in 1948, passed a resolution favouring state-aided, contributory health insurance. The plan would include every resident of the province and be administered by an independent, non-political commission. The medical profession would be represented on the commission by members elected by the College, and doctors would be paid on a fee-for-service basis.

In the same year a voluntary, prepaid medical care plan began to offer both medical and surgical services by medically qualified practitioners in Nova Scotia. The Medical Society of that province had established the plan itself in order to prevent the imposition of a government-sponsored plan.

The CMA supported these plans, and in 1949 issued a Statement of Policy on health insurance which recommended the extension of voluntary plans. The government, it was proposed, would pay the premiums for those who could not afford them. Additional services would be added to the plan in stages, the first and most important being the coverage of every Canadian for the costs of hospital services. Most of the costs would be met by payments from individuals. The government would only cover contributions for indigent people.

The CMA executive, concerned that government health programs threatened professional autonomy and widened East-West regional disparity, moved to consolidate

[f] For more on J.J. Heagerty, the Heagerty Committee, and the federal government's health care plans during World War II, see Heather McDougall, "Into Thin Air: Making National Health Policy, 1939–45," *Canadian Bulletin of Medical History* 26, no. 2 (2009): 283–313.

its dominance of the provincial associations. In 1950 it amalgamated the positions of General Secretary and Managing Editor of the *Journal*. Dr. T.C. Routley assumed both positions, and the *Journal* became an explicit tool for the Association to dictate to the provincial medical associations and to control any actions proposed by them.

In 1951 the CMA amalgamated independent health insurance agencies in all the provinces under its control. The so-called Trans-Canada Medical Plan was a national organization which became a political alternative to state-aided plans.

In 1953 the CMA's Committee on Economics began a study of health insurance plans. After two years the General Council adopted a statement on health insurance in Canada, outlining the CMA's role if and when the government brought in universal health insurance. Throughout the statement, the Association emphasized the profession's autonomy and dominance in the practice of medicine.[26]

The CMA wanted any health insurance programs to be an extension of existing prepaid medical insurance plans such as the Trans-Canada Plan.[27] It wanted to set up a Department of Public Health to provide preventative services. The opportunity of insuring for medical services would be available to every Canadian, including dependents. Only thus, the Canadian Medical Association believed, would the highest standards of health services—preventative, curative, and rehabilitative—be achieved. There would be a balanced development of diagnostic facilities, general hospitals, rehabilitative centres, chronic care facilities, and home care programs. Health insurance would be administered by an independent, non-political commission representative of those who were providing and receiving the services.

The CMA recommended that provincial governments collaborate in the administrative and financial task of extending health insurance to those not covered by existing voluntary medical care plans, leaving to each community the responsibility for maintaining environmental and workplace safety, and for providing preventative services. Hospitals, health departments, and all other health agencies would co-ordinate their activities to provide their services effectively and economically. Hospital location, facilities, and size would be planned on a regional basis. Alternate and professional organizations and government health agencies would participate in community and provincial health planning. Health insurance legislation would be preceded by consultation with the organized medical profession and other affected groups. The various services would be introduced in planned stages.

In the 1950s, the Ontario Medical Association and the Saskatchewan College of Physicians and Surgeons took different positions in the health insurance debate. The Saskatchewan College did not have a comprehensive policy statement of its own, but passed resolutions supportive of CMA policy. The OMA formulated its own policy, which diverged somewhat from that of the CMA. The OMA maintained, for instance, that it should determine its own method of remuneration in any health insurance plan, and that it was only the profession that could determine the quality of care.[28] It urged the government to let the people of Ontario decide, 1) whether they wished to prepay the costs of medical services, and, if so, whether prepayment would be voluntary or mandatory, and 2) the degree of government intervention in any plan.

Nevertheless, OMA and CMA policies were congruent in several key aspects: they each agreed that the profession should control the practice of medicine, that there should be a free doctor-patient relationship, that the administration of any government-sponsored plan should be by an independent commission with a balanced membership of those providing and those receiving the services, that education and research programs be separated from service programs in administration and funding, that working conditions and remuneration be such that the profession of medicine would continue to attract sufficient personnel of high enough calibre, and that medication and arbitration boards be established representative of those giving, receiving, and administering the service.

The Saskatchewan College of Physicians and Surgeons consequently passed a resolution in favour of state-aided, contributory health insurance. The plan would include every resident of the province, be administered by an independent, non-political commission, and the medical profession would be represented on the commission by members elected by the College. The profession, again, would be paid on a fee-for-service basis.

In April 1953 the College submitted a brief to the Health Services Planning Commission which records its recommendations. The College agreed that a comprehensive health insurance plan should be established at the earliest possible date, providing the plan conformed with the 1949 CMA policy statement.

In 1959, however, at the College's annual meeting in Saskatoon, a resolution was passed which recommended the extension of health and sickness benefits through indemnity and service plans. The College thus reversed its earlier position and declared itself opposed to a government-controlled, province-wide medical care plan.

Both the Saskatchewan College of Physicians and Surgeons and the Canadian Medical Association in 1959 favoured the extension of contributory health insurance encompassing the principle of pre-payment. The opportunity to pre-pay for medical care would be voluntary and available to every Canadian. The College and the CMA both emphasized that any plan must provide the highest quality of medical care (as defined by the profession), with the responsibility for maintaining this care resting with the profession only. Improving the quality of services must not interfere with physicians' economic security. Professional education and research activities were the keys to high quality medical services.

The development of organized medicine in Canada and the United States demonstrates how health policies were formulated at the national level in both countries. The policies of provincial medical associations are controlled at the national level by the Canadian Medical Association, while the policies espoused by the CMA are significantly influenced by the interests of the medical profession in the United States. Thus, the Saskatchewan profession's hostility to government-sponsored medical insurance and the community clinic movement arose from, and was strongly supported by, the North American medical establishment.

This professional body's hostility to state intervention in the health system in both the United States and Canada was and continues to be based on physician remuneration. Fee-for-service payment allows doctors to control their incomes. Under it they can increase their cash flow simply by increasing their patient load. With salaried service, on the other hand, doctors cannot gain financially by taking less time with each patient and thereby fitting more patients into the working day. Under salaried medical service, patient care, not the pressure to make more money, is the priority.

The CMA continues to argue that third party involvement in the financing of health care interferes with the professional freedom of doctors.

Notes

1. George M. Torrance, "Socio-historical Overview" in D'Arcy Coburn and Torrance New (eds.), *Health and Canadian Society* (Toronto: Fitzhenry and Whiteside Ltd, 1981), 15.

2. E. Richard Brown, "He Who Pays the Piper: Foundations of the Medical Profession and Medical Education Reform," *International Journal of Health Services* 10, no. 1 (1980).

3. E. Richard Brown, "Public Health in Imperialism: Early Rockefeller Programs at Home and Abroad" in John Ehrenreich (ed.), *The Cultural Crisis of Modern Medicine* (New York: Monthly Review Press, 1978).

4. Donald Creighton, *Canada's First Century* (Toronto: MacMillan of Canada, 1970).

5. Ibid., 102.

6. Ibid.

7. Brown, "He Who Pays the Piper..."

8. C. David Naylor, *Private Practice, Public Payment: Canadian Medicine and the Politics of Health Insurance, 1911–1966* (Montreal: McGill-Queens University Press, 1986).

9. Ibid.

10. Richard Carter, *The Doctor Business* (New York: Doubleday and Company Inc., 1958).

11. Canadian Medical Association, *Journal* 84 (March 1961).

12. Saskatchewan Department of Public Health, "Selected Briefs to the Advisory Planning Committee on Medical Care," Vol. 1 (1961).

13. John Ehrenreich and Barbara Ehrenreich, *The American Health Empire: Power, Profits and Politics* (Toronto: Random House of Canada Ltd, 1970), 127.

14. Ibid., 159.

15. Carter, *The Doctor Business*, 51.

16. Daniel S. Hirschfield, *The Lost Reform: The Campaign for Compulsory Health Insurance in the United States from 1932 to 1943* (Massachusetts: Harvard University Press, 1970), 44.

17. Ibid., 85.

18. Ibid., 44.

19. Ibid., 90.

20. Ibid., 97.

21. Carter, *The Doctor Business*, 201.

22. Ibid., 210.

23. Ehrenreich and Ehrenreich, *The American Health Empire*, 129.

24. Naylor, *Private Practice, Public Payment.*

25. Canadian Medical Association, *Journal* 87 (September 1962).

26. David Coburn, George Torrance, and Joseph Kaufert, "Medical Dominance in Canada in Historical Perspective: The Rise and Fall Of Medicine," *International Journal of Health Services* 13, no. 1 (1983).

27. Government of Saskatchewan, "Advisory Planning Briefs."

28. Naylor, *Private Practice, Public Payment.*

Chapter 3
A Brief History of Compulsory Universal Health Insurance

Federal assistance to the hospital plan commenced in 1958, and the CCF proceeded toward its goal of creating a comprehensive, universal medical care plan. In April 1959 a committee was struck by Cabinet to develop proposals for the plan, and was instructed to report back within the year. If its recommendations were acceptable, a public committee would be established to discuss them.

At its annual meeting in October 1959, the Saskatchewan College of Physicians and Surgeons made known its opposition to any government-controlled, province-wide medical care plan. They supported instead an "extension of health and sickness benefits through indemnity and service plans."[1] The physicians feared that government intervention would reduce their own influence and autonomy. The CCF, on the other hand, was committed to a province-wide plan, and in 1960 Premier Douglas made the government's intentions clear:

> The Government of Saskatchewan is convinced that the time has arrived when we can establish a prepaid medical care plan in our march toward comprehensive health insurance that will cover all our people and will ensure a high standard of medical care to every citizen of Saskatchewan.[2]

This announcement diverged somewhat from the proposals set out by the Cabinet committee, which had stressed the importance of a unified health service that included preventative and rehabilitative care as well as medical care. In the announcement, Douglas outlined the basic principles of the plan:

> 1. The pre-payment principle—that medical care should be paid for on an insurance basis;
>
> 2. Universal coverage—it must cover every person in the province;
>
> 3. High quality of service—the plan's major objective would be improvement of quality, distribution, and availability of care;
>
> 4. The plan should be government sponsored, administered by the Department of Public Health, responsible to the Legislature and the people of the province through the Minister of Public Health;
>
> 5. The plan should be acceptable both to those providing the service and those receiving it.[3]

Before proceeding, the government appointed an Advisory Planning Committee on Medical Care to recommend the best methods of developing a program in keeping with the principles outlined by Premier Douglas.

Negotiations between the government and the doctors began on December 30, 1959, when the Minister of Public Health wrote to the College of Physicians and Surgeons inviting the College to name three representatives to the Advisory Planning Committee. He included draft terms of reference for the committee with his letter. The College replied on January 18, 1960, objecting to the committee's mandate. They felt that any decisions regarding the quality of medical services were best made by the profession itself. Outside interference, whether from the government or a public committee, could only be detrimental. The College refused to participate on the Advisory Planning Committee and instead began to lobby for political and public support of their position. They eventually spent close to $90,000 in their efforts to defeat the CCF and its medicare plan. Opposition parties sided with the doctors, weakening the position of the CCF. Accordingly, the mandate of the committee was changed.

The revised mandate gave the Advisory Planning Committee the authority to study a medical care insurance program for the province and to report on public needs in other health fields.[4] It limited the committee's activities to studying existing plans and removed the possibility of a critical evaluation of medical services. The committee could not, for example, assess the benefits of medical care in relation to alternative forms of health care. This clearly served the interests of physicians, as it ensured that their control over medical practice would remain unchallenged. For the government, the revised mandate represented an opportunity to carry through with their promise to provide prepaid medical care to the people of Saskatchewan. The Minister of Health wrote to the College of Physicians and Surgeons:

> The Government's position is that the nature of any program which might be introduced should wait on the advice and recommendation of the Committee which is being set up. The advice will be given I believe only after the Committee has been able to make a thorough study of all the diverse issues involved. The Committee cannot be bound to accept the views of the Government without study, nor can the committee be bound to accept the views of the College without similar study.[5]

On March 29, 1960, Dr. A.J. Davies, then College president, wrote to Premier Douglas and announced the appointment of three physicians as representatives on the Advisory Planning Committee. The other nine members included three representatives from the Government of Saskatchewan, one from the Saskatchewan Federation of Labour, one from the Chamber of Commerce, one from the College of Medicine, and two representatives of the public. Dr. W.P. Thompson,[a] a former president of the University of Saskatchewan, was appointed chairperson.

On April 26, the terms of reference for the Advisory Planning Committee were approved by Order-in-Council. These terms limited the Committee's role to that of

[a] The Advisory Planning Committee would become popularly known as the Thompson Committee. Walter Palmer Thompson was originally a plant geneticist educated at Harvard. Shortly after he retired as president of the University of Saskatchewan, he was asked by Premier Tommy Douglas to chair the committee that would provide advice to the government on how best to implement medicare. From the beginning, the Thompson Committee was divided between the members representing organized medicine and its allies and those who supported the principle of universal medical care insurance.

implementing a medical care insurance program. The medical profession maintained its dominance in matters such as doctor-patient relationships, professional judgement, education, and research. This restricted the committee to financial and administrative matters, and prevented any infringement of the medical profession's autonomy.[6]

The Advisory Planning Committee began its deliberation on May 9. It considered briefs from 49 organizations, conducted 33 public and seven private hearings, and examined medical care plans in seven foreign countries.

In December the College of Physicians and Surgeons presented its brief to the Committee. The brief urged that those patients "judged to be able to pay for medical service insurance should be encouraged to participate in the excellent programs available through prepaid plans and licensed insurance companies. It is the responsibility of democratic government to assist those in society who are unable to obtain medical care insurance."[7] The College concluded that a single method of insurance, compulsory for all and controlled by government, would result in inferior service at a higher cost.

The brief acknowledged the presence of various minority opinions within the profession. Some physicians, for instance, did not believe insurance was desirable because doctors had always taken the economic circumstances of their patients into consideration when billing for their services. The introduction of insurance, they considered, would terminate a responsibility the profession had traditionally assumed. A second minority opinion was held by some physicians who were familiar with the Swift Current Medical Plan. They supported the introduction of compulsory service on a local basis, they said, as long as government control was not instituted. They opposed any attempt to abrogate local policymaking and administrative autonomy by centralizing control of the whole province in any one agency. This position reiterates the two principles commonly upheld by Saskatchewan people: co-operative action at the community level. The College, in any case, downplayed these minority opinions and took the position that the proper role of government was to assist only those in need.

The Saskatchewan Farmers' Union brief to the Advisory Planning Committee supported the concept of a government-sponsored medical care plan with the following provisions: the plan must be universal; there must be uniformity of care for everyone in the province; the plan must not be administered in any way by private health schemes; there must be no deterrent fees of any kind; in isolated areas, visits by medical specialists should be encouraged by offering salaried service; research and preventative health care must be encouraged; doctors may practice outside the plan, but at the patient's expense.[8]

The Saskatchewan Federation of Labour also supported a universal, comprehensive medical care plan. Its brief to the Committee opposed private health schemes as well as deterrent fees. It wanted the plan to be administered through a branch of government that would co-ordinate all existing and proposed health services, and stressed the need for the Department of Public Health to upgrade its programs. Physicians were to be remunerated on a salary basis to guard against abuses of the system which fee-for-service payments might encourage. The SFL strongly supported group medical practices and community health centres, and suggested that there be an advisory council and an appeals procedure available to all.[9]

Several of the briefs presented to the Committee described the advantages and disadvantages of health schemes already in operation in Saskatchewan. A brief from the Swift Current Health Region suggested that the province be divided into seven regions, each administering its own plan. Patients would be eligible for service if they were residents in a region and if they had paid an insurance premium. The plan would thus be financed through patient fees and government support. Physicians would be paid on a fee-for-service contract through the College of Physicians and Surgeons.

The Group Medical Services brief supported a voluntary insurance scheme, suggesting that group contracts be awarded to local areas and that each area be responsible for the administration of its own plan. Local authorities would decide who was able to pay premiums, and the government would provide financial assistance to those who could not. Both the GMS and the Swift Current Health Region proposals attempted to make health care community based, but they did not address the key issues of universality and accessibility.

On July 9, 1961, the College of Physicians and Surgeons presented a supplementary submission to the Advisory Planning Committee; it constituted a formal response to the various proposals which had been received by the Committee. The College stated emphatically that fees for services rendered was the only acceptable method of remunerating doctors. It opposed the idea of group practice, stressing that physicians should have the right to select the type and location of their practices, and it re-stated its position on insurance:

> a) ...self-supporting citizens should be encouraged to insure themselves and their families by subscribing to one of the voluntary programs of Medical Services Insurance.
>
> b) ...three elements of the population require assistance from public funds to permit them to obtain the Medical Services Insurance they require: those persons of low income of all ages, those persons over 65 years whose premiums require subsidy, and those who are uninsurable at regular rates because of pre-existing conditions.[10]

On September 25, 1961, the Advisory Planning Committee released its Interim Report, recommending the implementation of a universal, comprehensive medical care plan administered by a public commission responsible to the Legislature through the Minister of Public Health. The three representatives from the College of Physicians and Surgeons and the representative from the Chamber of Commerce opposed these recommendations and submitted a Minority Report. In it, they questioned the need for a universal plan and proposed instead that government subsidies be paid to non-government carriers for persons unable to finance their own premiums. Such a system, they claimed, would achieve the desired universality, provide for more than a single carrier, avoid the undesirable feature of compulsion, and permit the practice of medicine to develop the highest standards of personal health care.

A Dissenting Report was submitted by Walter Smishek,[b] representing the

[b] Walter Smishek was a prominent trade unionist in Saskatchewan who was executive secretary of the Saskatchewan Federation of Labour and served on the political action committee of the Canadian Labour Congress. In 1964, Smishek entered politics. He won his constituency (Regina East) and would remain in the Saskatchewan Legislature until 1982. He served as Minister of Health (1971–75) and Minister of Finance (1975–79) in the Blakeney government and was most known for the introduction of a universal prescription drug plan and a children's dental program. Smishek also replaced fee-for-service funding with global funding for community clinics shortly after becoming Minister of Health.

Saskatchewan Federation of Labour. Mr. Smishek opposed the majority recommendations on four items: he stated a preference for administration by the Department of Public Health rather than by an independent commission; he did not agree that fee for service should be the major method of payment; he registered his objection to utilization fees and to direct personal premiums.

Premier Douglas pushed ahead with the majority recommendations of the Interim Report. On October 25, 1961, he introduced the Medical Care Insurance Bill at a special session of the Legislature. At its annual meeting in October, the College of Physicians and Surgeons passed resolutions opposing the main features of the Bill. On November 17, the Saskatchewan Medical Care Insurance Act was enacted and given assent. In its final stages, the Act was piloted through the Legislature by Premier W.S. Lloyd, who had taken over after Douglas resigned in November to assume federal leadership of the New Democratic Party.

The Saskatchewan Medical Care Insurance Act, 1961, provided that everyone who had been a resident of Saskatchewan for three months or longer, and who had registered with the Medical Care Plan, was eligible for benefits, including specialist services when the patient was referred by the family doctor. The Act also ensured the free choice of doctors.

The Medical Care Insurance Commission was appointed on January 9, 1962, with Mr. D.D. Tansley[c] as Chairperson. Other members included: Dr. O.K. Hjertaas[d] from the Prince Albert Community Clinic as Vice-Chairperson, Mr. A.V. Kipling from Melfort, Mr. S. Robertson from Swift Current, Mr. G. Taylor[e] from Saskatoon, and Dr. Samuel Wolfe from Saskatoon. The Commission met for the first time on January 15, and immediately concentrated on three principal tasks: setting up administrative machinery, establishing links with the medical profession, and formulating policy within the framework of the Act.

The College of Physicians and Surgeons declined all invitations to participate in the Commission's work on the grounds that the profession wanted nothing to do with the Act or anything proceeding from it. For the same reason, the College declined

[c] Donald D. Tansley was a senior public servant in the Douglas government. He worked under A.W. Johnson in the Treasury department until 1960 when he became executive director of the Government Finance Office. He accepted the job only after Premier Lloyd was unable to find anyone outside the government willing to take the job. Convinced that a doctors' strike was virtually unavoidable, Tansley was most responsible for convincing Lloyd and his cabinet to allow the Medical Care Insurance Commission to recruit doctors in the United Kingdom (Saskatchewan Archives Board, Regina, R-8463 to R-8464, transcript of interview of Don Tansley by Jean Larmour, Feb. 10, 1982).

[d] Graduating in 1942, Orville Hjertaas practiced medicine in rural Saskatchewan until joining the Health Service Planning Commission as a health region organizer in 1945. Months later, he became secretary of the Commission, and then joined two fellow University of Manitoba classmates in establishing a general practice in Prince Albert, Saskatchewan. When medicare was introduced in 1961–62, Hjertaas found that he and his partners were on opposite sides of the question, and he soon organized the community clinic in Prince Albert. See Stuart Houston and Bill Waiser, *Tommy's Team: The People Behind the Douglas Years* (Markham, ON: Fifth House, 2010), 60–65.

[e] A committed socialist and veteran of the Spanish Civil War, George Taylor was a Saskatoon lawyer and active supporter of the community clinic movement.

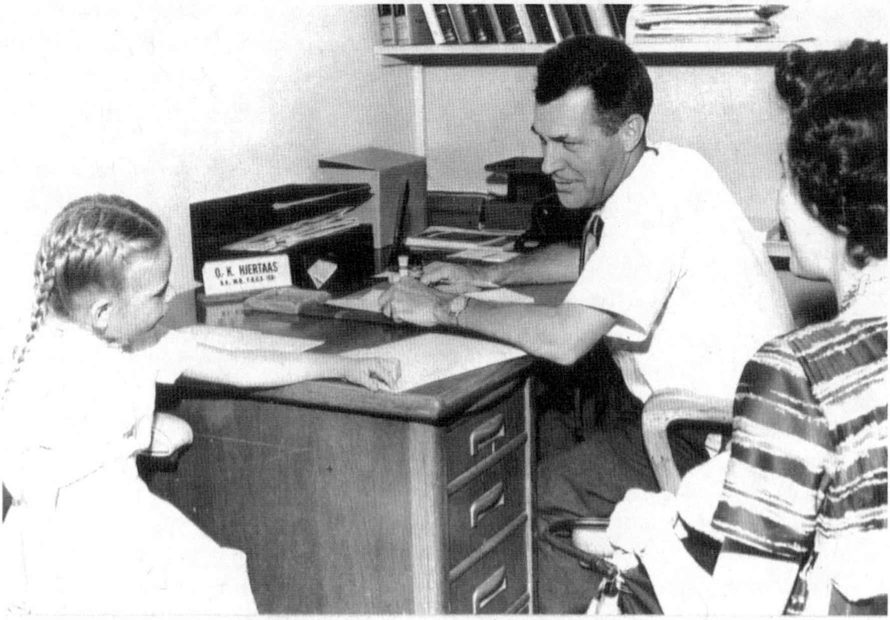

Dr. Orville Hjertaas, member of the Medical Care Insurance Commission and founder of the Prince Albert Community Clinic (Prince Alberta Community Clinic, photo #19-PA).

subsequent invitations to discuss the implications of the Act and plans for its implementation. In fact, the College had no communication with the Commission until May, 1962.[11]

The date set by the government for the commencement of medicare was April 1, 1962, but by late February it was clear that this was insufficient time to complete the administrative planning and to assemble and train staff. On the advice of the Commission, the government set the date ahead to July 1. The College of Physicians and Surgeons met with the Cabinet on March 28, reiterating the proposal it had made earlier to the Thompson Committee. At another meeting, on April 1, the College advanced an eight-point proposal as its final concession:

> 1) That medical care insurance be province-wide and universally available to all Saskatchewan residents on the payment of a premium;
>
> 2) That this be made available through existing or new voluntary prepaid agencies;
>
> 3) That a Registration Board function as an approved body for these insurance agencies;
>
> 4) That government would pay the entire premium for persons deemed to be indigent;
>
> 5) That the government would provide, as a subsidy, a stated number of dollars for each contract offered by approved agencies;
>
> 6) That each approved agency would determine the amount of money required in addition to the subsidy, and would charge this

additional amount as a premium to be paid by subscribers who enrol on a voluntary basis;

7) That patients would pay their accounts directly to their doctors and would obtain from their approved agency a refund of a major portion of the expense incurred;

8) That the profession would not make charges to the indigent groups in excess of the amount of refund to which the patient is entitled.[12]

This proposal was rejected on April 11. The government objected to the suggestion that patients pay doctors directly, as this would discourage people from seeking medical care, and the key objectives of the insurance plan—accessibility and universality—would be compromised. The government also objected to forcing indigent persons to identify themselves when they sought medical care, as this might subject them to discrimination or prejudice. Finally, the government objected to the suggestion that public money be turned over to private insurance agencies; this would increase administrative costs because of the multiplicity of agencies competing for the public dollar. The government suggested instead that sections of the Act be revised to achieve the following:

1) Remove concern about the possible interference with professional standards and professional independence;

2) Provide for a mechanism by which physician's remuneration could be arrived at in a fair and equitable manner, including a specific appeals procedure;

3) Provide for appeal methods for the disposition of all differences on the part of physicians respecting the administration of the Act or cases of alleged interference;

4) Provide for regional bodies to assess and review accounts where these become the subject of dispute;

5) Provide, if desired, for an arrangement whereby a member of the profession designated by the College would overview administrative matters affecting individual physicians;

6) Permit the appointment, in consultation with the College, of additional members to the Medical Care Insurance Commission.[13]

The College rejected these proposals, and the meetings ended without agreement. Premier Lloyd announced the government's intention to proceed with the plan provided for in the Medical Care Insurance Act. On April 14, the Legislature amended the Act to permit the Commission to act as agent of a beneficiary in any matter related to the payment of a bill. The amended Act contained an "opting-out" provision which allowed physicians to declare that they did not want the Commission to act as an agent in the payment of accounts, and it provided that other government agencies paying for medical care could arrange for the Medical Care Insurance Commission to act as paymaster. It also provided protection to physicians, so that no action could be taken against them on the basis of particulars given to the Commission for payment of insured services. The Act further stipulated that, in the event of a dispute over rates of payment, either the Commission or the profession could refer the matter to a mediation board.

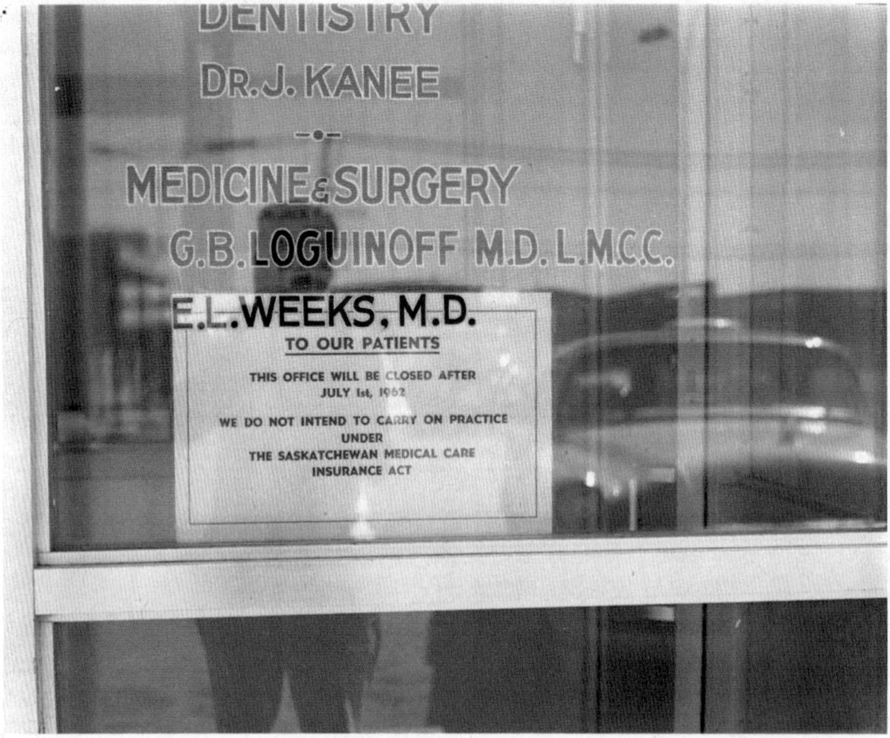

Closure of a doctor's office during the 1962 strike (SAB Photographic Services Series, R-PS62-229, photo #10).

The College of Physicians and Surgeons continued to speak out against the government. On May 3, it met in a special session in Regina. Premier Lloyd addressed the meeting, at his own request:

> If the government promised that a plan must be acceptable to doctors we also promised that it must be acceptable to patients. Following this thinking we promised that a plan would incorporate the prepayment principle; we promised that it would cover every person in the province; we promised a high quality of care and we promised that any plan would be administered by the Department of Public Health. We sincerely believe that we have gone some distance in trying to devise a plan which would be acceptable to doctors and not violate the other principles. We are prepared at all times to consider sincere requests for changes in matters which cause the profession legitimate concern. My request is that a fair trial for the plan is the only test of acceptability.[14]

The College maintained its opposition, feeling that the plan would severely restrict the activities of physicians, and that it would lead to salaried service, turning medical professionals into employees. Physicians wanted no interference with their activities and no reduction in their autonomy. When the government refused to capitulate, the College increased its pressure with public meetings, by lobbying opposition parties, and

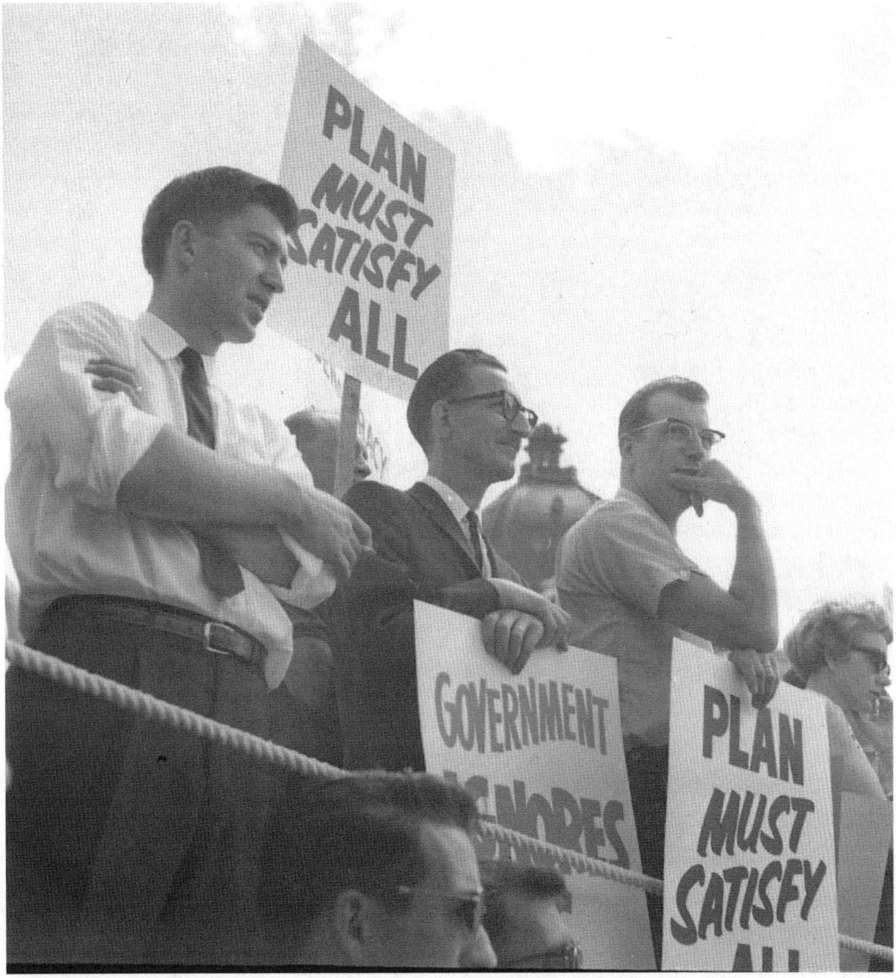

Photo taken at the anti-medicare rally on July 11, 1962 (SAB Photographic Services Series, R-PS62-229, photo #19).

by advertising the supposed consequences of the plan to their patients. Public support for the physicians was mounting. People feared that their doctors would leave the province and they would be left with no medical care. The College announced that, if the Medical Care Plan came into effect, doctors would withdraw normal services and provide free emergency services in a limited number of hospitals across the province.

The government was increasingly concerned at the threatened withdrawal of physicians' services. Rural areas were particularly vulnerable because of long distances to the cities and an already short supply of doctors. The rural vote was important to the government; farmers constituted a large proportion of its support. Premier Lloyd attempted to reassure doctors that the government had no intention of changing or challenging the physician's role in the health system:

> In prescribing medical treatment your knowledge and your word are supreme. The government has no wish or intention to change or

> challenge that supremacy. … Medical services are essential to health and to life itself. Good medical services are part of the basis for a healthy, productive economy.[15]

In June the Commission undertook an emergency program to recruit doctors for temporary service. From June 22 to 25, the government and the College met in Regina. The government offered to allow doctors to bill patients directly, and patients would then be reimbursed by the Commission. This was not acceptable, the College responded, unless the Act itself was completely rewritten. The meetings concluded without agreement. On June 27, the government announced that physicians were to have the option of billing patients rather than the Commission.

On July 1, 1962, the Medical Care Plan came into effect, and most physicians in Saskatchewan withdrew normal services [the community clinics, which had been recruiting staff throughout the crisis, continued to offer medical care]. The College of Physicians and Surgeons announced that emergency services would be available at 29 hospitals across the province. Throughout the first half of July, the College maintained its position that a settlement could be reached only with the withdrawal of the Medical Care Insurance Act. Certain municipal councils passed resolutions against the plan. Some hospital boards denied privileges to doctors who came to help during the emergency. The College increased its pressure by becoming specific as to who could obtain a license to practice medicine in the province, and by harassing physicians who had been recruited by the Commission. "Keep Our Doctors" committees, established with the financial support of the College and the Saskatchewan Liberal Party to pressure the government to rescind the Act, organized a rally on July 11 at the Legislature in Regina. Liberal leader Ross Thatcher was the principal speaker.

On July 16, Lord Stephen Taylor,[f] a British doctor who had participated in the planning of the National Health Service in the United Kingdom, arrived in Regina to assume the role of mediator in the negotiations between the government and the College. On July 18, Dr. Harold Dalgleish, President of the College of Physicians and Surgeons, addressed the CCF-NDP Annual Convention in Saskatoon, stating that the College had dropped its demand that the Saskatchewan Medical Care Insurance Act be suspended before discussion with the government could be resumed. Negotiations commenced from that day until 12:45 pm, July 23, when Lord Taylor announced that an agreement had been reached.

[f] Stephen Taylor was a physician and member of the Labour Party. As one of the few physicians supporting the idea of a universal health system, he assisted in the development of the Labour government's blueprint for what would become the National Health Service. After losing his seat in 1950, he worked as a health administrator and consultant, and was made life peer (Baron Taylor) in 1958. In 1962, he acted as a go-between in the final days of the doctors' strike and as the catalyst for the Saskatoon Agreement, the compromise that ended the strike. See Geoffrey Rivett, "Taylor, Stephen James Lake, Baron Taylor (1910–1988)," *Oxford Dictionary of National Biography* (Oxford: Oxford University Press, 2007), accessed July 10, 2010: http://www.oxforddnb.com/view/article/39545; Allan Blakeney, *An Honourable Calling: Political Memoirs* (Toronto: University of Toronto Press, 2008), 60–62. For Stephen's own account of his intervention in Saskatchewan, see his autobiography, *A Natural History of Everyday Life* (Cambridge: The Memoir Club, 1988), 341–89.

Notes

1. Interdepartmental Committee to Study Medical Care Insurance, "Organized Medicine's Official Position on Health Insurance" (1959), 8.

2. T.C. Douglas, "More Abundant Living," Debate on the Speech from the Throne (Regina: Saskatchewan Legislature, 1960).

3. W.S. Lloyd, "Financing the Medical Care Program," Address in the Saskatchewan Legislature, Special Session (October 20, 1961).

4. Saskatchewan Department of Public Health, "Selected Briefs to the Advisory Planning Committee on Medical Care," Vol. 1 (1961).

5. Ibid.

6. Government of Saskatchewan, "Interim Report of the Advisory Planning Committee on Medical Care" (1961).

7. Advisory Planning Briefs.

8. Ibid.

9. Ibid.

10. Ibid.

11. Lloyd, "Financing the Medical Care Program," 6.

12. Ibid., 7.

13. Ibid., 8.

14. Ibid., 11.

15. Ibid., 15.

Chapter 4
The Saskatoon Agreement

Throughout the summer of 1962, community health associations were formed across the province with the intention of establishing local clinics. In only a few places had the possibility even been discussed before the doctors withdrew their services on July 1. By September 30, however, a provincial association of community clinics had 22 affiliated associations with paid-up memberships of 7,652 families. Fifteen other associations, not yet affiliated, reported memberships totalling 3,500. It was estimated that these 37 community associations had family memberships totalling over 12,000, representing more than 40,000 people.

The provincial co-ordinating committee had been established in July 1962. This was followed by the election of a permanent board of directors at the first provincial convention in November of that year. A permanent provincial office was established and a staff hired:

> **Executive Director:** Stanley Rands, formerly deputy director of psychiatric services with the provincial government. In addition to giving overall direction to the work of the association, the Executive Director was responsible for the doctor recruitment program and doctor allocation, relations between local associations and doctors, and relations between the Community Health Services Association, governments, and other health agencies.
>
> **Executive Assistant:** Maynard Woollard, former high school teacher and advertising executive. Mr. Woollard was primarily responsible for community organization, finances, public and community information, and health education and related activities.
>
> **Clinic Consultant:** Thomas Ludwig, formerly with the National Farmers Union (USA) on the development of rural co-ops, the Mineworkers Welfare and Retirement Fund as a clinic consultant, and the Centerville group of clinics (Pennsylvania) as assistant clinic administrator. Mr. Ludwig was responsible for the physical setup of the clinics, administrative and accounting procedures, staff training, and related matters.
>
> **Medical Consultant:** Samuel Wolfe,[a] MD, MPH, DrPH, medical director of the Saskatoon Community Clinic and a member of the

[a] Sam Wolfe (1923–93) received his medical degree in Toronto in 1950. He then moved to Porcupine Plain, Saskatchewan, where he worked as a family physician. After receiving a Rockefeller

Medical Care Insurance Commission. Dr. Wolfe was the chief advisor to the provincial association in all matters relating to physicians and the practice of medicine. He also gave assistance, when required, to other clinic doctors.

Chief Recruiting Officer: Terence Gardiner, MA, MRCS, LRCP, was responsible for the recruitment of physicians in the United Kingdom and elsewhere overseas.

These were the minimum of positions required to direct the development of community clinics to their full potential in a co-operative manner. Once clinics were established and playing their part fully in a successful Medical Care Plan, it was anticipated that the costs of the central office would be borne by the clinics.

The extent of the activity of this board and its affiliated local associations was indicated in a survey carried out in mid-March, 1963, nine months after the organizing had begun.[1] At that stage, local associations were concentrating on raising money and providing facilities. Biggar, with 600 family memberships, had raised over $40,000 in member loans, had purchased a building, and was preparing it for a maximum of five doctors. Estevan had 300 family members, three doctors working in a rented facility, and was going ahead with plans for constructing its own building. Moose Jaw, with almost 900 family memberships, had rented facilities adequate for three doctors and had two doctors practising. Nipawin had a three-doctor clinic in operation; two had been practising there before July 1, 1962, and were in the process of turning the premises over to the association, which was planning to enlarge them and rent them back to the doctors.

North Battleford had almost 700 family members and facilities for three doctors, with one practising. Prince Albert, with 1,200 family members and five doctors working in rented premises, was planning a $240,000 clinic with facilities for 12 doctors, two dentists, a laboratory, and a pharmacy. The Regina Association's 1,700 family members had provided $50,000 to cover initial operating expenses and to purchase equipment. Similarly, Saskatoon's 1,400 family members had raised approximately $50,000, mainly in the form of personal loans. The association was renting premises, and re-renting them to the medical group of six doctors and support staff. The Watrous Association, with a membership of 325 families, had raised $17,000 from members, spent $9,000 on a building, and allotted the remainder to the initial period of deficit financing. One physician began practising in March 1963; a second was expected the following month.

Three other communities had provided premises and rented them to doctors, but had to close when the doctors left: Weyburn with 500 family members, Wynyard with 450, and Radville with nearly 400.

Seven additional communities were ready for doctors in March 1963. Assiniboia,

scholarship, he completed his doctorate in public health at Columbia University in 1961. He returned to Saskatchewan to take up a post at the medical school, and was subsequently appointed by the government to the Medical Care Insurance Commission. In 1962, in the wake of the doctors' strike, he resigned from the University of Saskatchewan and became the Saskatoon community clinic's first medical director: see John Bury, "Wolfe, Sam" in *The Encyclopedia of Saskatchewan* (Regina: Canadian Plains Research Center, 2005), 1016–17. With co-author Robin F. Badgley, Sam Wolfe wrote the one and only major account of the events of 1962 entitled, *Doctors' Strike: Medical Care and Conflict in Saskatchewan* (Toronto: Macmillan of Canada, 1967).

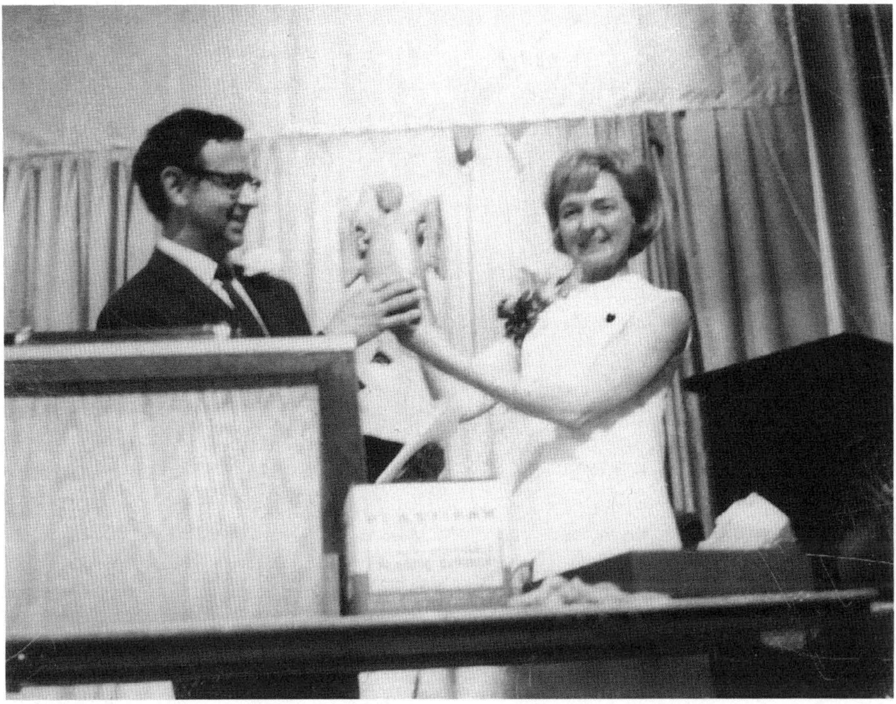

Dr. Sam Wolfe, seen here with his wife, Mary (Saskatoon Community Clinic, photo #16-SK).

with almost 400 family members, had purchased a lot on the main street and was intending to build a $40,000 clinic; meanwhile, they rented premises. Eston had already built a $40,000 clinic capable of accommodating four doctors, a dentist, a laboratory, and a pharmacy; this building had been ready since February, and $35,000 had been raised from the members. Kamsack had rented a building and planned to start remodelling for a clinic early in April. Kindersley had purchased temporary facilities for $12,500, and planned to construct a building similar to the one in Eston the following year. Kinistino, too, had secured facilities and was planning to build a new clinic the following year. Lloydminster was remodelling a building to suit the needs of its clinic. Melfort also had acquired a building and was prepared to remodel and add to it as soon as physician services could be provided.

An additional 15 communities had organized health associations, but held back from further commitments because of the expense and growing uncertainty about whether doctors would be available. Though cautious, these associations anticipated no trouble in securing facilities once doctors became available. Two other communities had done some initial organizing, but by March 1963 no association had yet been formed.

The situation was summarized in the Community Health Services Association brief to the government in March 1963:

> • Almost 15,000 families, representing approximately 50,000 people, in 36 areas of the province have joined the community clinic movement, with thousands of others signifying their support in one form or another.

- Thirty-four areas have formed active associations.
- Eight associations have purchased or built clinic premises.
- Eleven associations have secured rented premises.
- Fifteen associations planned to rent, buy, or build facilities, depending on circumstances at the time doctors became available.
- Over $325,000 has been raised through memberships, donations, and loans of various kinds.
- Three associations which were renting in March 1963 were developing plans to build. These projects would involve the expenditure of an additional $375,000.
- Additional expenditures by other associations were expected to involve the spending of up to another half-million dollars in the year ahead.[2]

These details demonstrate the vigour and tenacity of the movement in proceeding with matters such as raising money and providing premises and equipment. But along with these tangible forward steps came changes of a different kind: in the attitudes of doctors and consumers, in new kinds of working relationships between professional people and association members, in the development of new types of health care programs.

In spite of the community action of those first nine months, however, at the end of March 1963 there were only nine clinics in operation, with a total of 24 doctors. Twenty other doctors had agreed to join clinic staffs, but a high dropout rate meant that not all of them could be counted on. A further 20 doctors were negotiating either with individual clinics or with the provincial association, but organizers felt even less confident that these prospects would materialize.

The slow progress in doctor recruitment was caused by the opposition of the medical profession, by provincial hospital policies, and by the Saskatoon Agreement.

On July 23, 1962, the Government of Saskatchewan and the Saskatchewan College of Physicians and Surgeons signed a memorandum of agreement in Saskatoon. The settlement, and the document itself, have come to be known as the Saskatoon Agreement.[3]

The settlement heralded the return of normal medical services. While Saskatchewan people generally were relieved at the news, some doctors were fearful that the agreement hadn't gone far enough to assuage their concerns. Many citizens, on the other hand, were concerned that the agreement had gone too far. This was especially the case in communities that were in the midst of developing clinics. But even they did not realize how far-reaching the impact of the settlement would be.

The Saskatoon Agreement effected significant changes to the medicare legislation—all of them concessions made by the Government of Saskatchewan in response to the demands of the medical profession. A number of the points agreed on were carried out by amending the Medical Care Insurance Act at a special session of the Legislature on August 2. Other issues were not dealt with by legislation, but remained points of agreement between the two parties. A third set of issues—issues relevant to the introduction of medicare and of deep concern to community clinics—was not touched upon either in the agreement or in the legislative amendments.

Through a legislative amendment, provisions for an Advisory Council and a Medical Advisory Committee were removed. It received little attention at the time, but the removal of the Committee emasculated the plan, changing it from a broad, publicly accountable health care system to a government-sponsored doctors' insurance plan. The Advisory Council was to have consisted of not more than 25 people who would mainly "be representatives of professional organizations whose members provide health services and of other organizations interested in a plan of medical care insurance for the residents of Saskatchewan."[4] The detail with which the structure and function of the Council were spelled out in the original legislation suggests that it was intended as a method of providing for continuing communication among the providers of health services, the beneficiaries of the plan, and the government.

Two members of the Advisory Council were to have been appointed by the government from the public at large, all others from nominees named by the various organizations of providers and consumers. The Council would have included representatives from the College of Physicians and Surgeons, the Saskatchewan Registered Nurses' Association, physiotherapists, hospital associations, farm organizations, trade unions, and the Community Health Services Association. It would have been available for advice to the Medical Care Insurance Commission, via the Minister of Health, on request. In addition, the Advisory Council would have been empowered to:

> propose improvements in, extensions of, restrictions with respect to, or modifications of, the medical care insurance plan...and submit any such proposals to the commission and to the minister. It would also have been authorized to obtain for the MCIC or other agencies "such information as is considered necessary with respect to the review and consideration of any aspect of the medical care insurance plan."[5]

Consultative bodies are not always useful. When appointed by governments they often do little more than run interference for the party in power, shielding it from the consequences of its actions, or inactions. In this case, however, since the members would have been nominated by organizations directly involved in issues concerning the new medicare plan, it might have exposed many situations which, in the absence of such a forum, festered in semi-darkness. Instances of discrimination by doctors and hospital boards, for instance, might have been brought into the open. Community clinics might have been able to get explanations for at least some of the baffling actions of the MCIC and the Health Department, explanations which were not available from bureaucrats or politicians. Community clinics would still have been handicapped by College opposition and lack of government support, but they would have been fighting with one arm tied rather than two.

In introducing the amendments in the Legislative Assembly on August 2, 1962, the Honourable W.G. Davies, then Minister of Public Health, stated:

> It was the opinion of the College of Physicians and Surgeons that there are existing methods of consultations and collaborations that can function in every way, as well as the Advisory Council that was mentioned in the present text of the bill. Moreover, it was felt that there would be to some extent a duplication in the present modes of consultation if the Advisory Council were to be created.[6]

E.A. Tollefson, author of *Bitter Medicine*, pointed out how unlikely it was that such "existing methods of consultations" would have been unknown to the persons responsible for the content of the legislation in the first place—the Deputy Minister of Public Health, for example. "It must be concluded," Tollefson observed, "that one or both of the parties to the Saskatoon Agreement did not want these bodies to exist."[7]

In view of the attitude of the College of Physicians and Surgeons toward health insurance and community clinics, it is not surprising that it would veto a proposal for citizen participation in the functioning of medicare. But the government, too, seemed leery of public participation in general and the community health associations in particular.

A second concession to the medical profession was the deletion of the "quality of care" clause. Implicit in the original legislation was the assumption that, since the Medical Care Insurance Commission was to be responsible for ensuring payment for medical care, it should also have some responsibility for ensuring that the quality of that care was satisfactory. Accordingly, Section 9 of the Act had authorized the Commission to "take such action as it considers necessary for the establishment and administration of a plan of medical care insurance for the residents of Saskatchewan and the improvement of the quality of the insured service provided under such a plan."[8]

The Saskatoon Agreement deleted all the words after "Saskatchewan." The result was that a public agency responsible for disbursing enormous sums of money could make no serious effort to guarantee that the money was well spent. Legal opinion holds that omission of the "quality of care" clause made little difference in practice, since it gave the Commission no powers not directly related to medical care insurance as such. While that is correct in the legal sense, there is good reason to believe that the phrase would have had a positive political effect. The Interdepartmental Committee to Study a Medical Care Program, for example, had recommended to Cabinet that the program include measures to encourage group practices. As the Committee pointed out, extensive experience and numerous studies have shown that patients are more likely to receive the best care when their doctors are working in regular consultation with their colleagues.[9]

In addition, "quality of care" can refer to many features of a medical service: preventative programs, a greater use of allied health personnel such as nurses and physiotherapists, transportation of the elderly and the poor to clinics, dietary counselling, and so on. Unfortunately, the deletion of the clause encouraged administrators to believe that they must do nothing which might displease the medical profession. Thus, an apparently minor change in legislation crippled the province's ability to encourage innovation in health services.

The Saskatoon Agreement also deleted Section 49—a second reference to the "quality of the services provided"—from the legislation. Section 49 had specified areas in which the MCIC might make regulations within the terms of the Medical Care Insurance Act and subject to the approval of the government. Clause 49(1), for example, had authorized regulations "respecting the maintenance and improvement of the quality of the services provided under this Act, to the end that the highest possible standard of service will be achieved."[10]

The medical profession's insistence on deleting the "quality of care" clauses is consistent with its long-term ambition to retain sole power over the definition and regulation of health care. The representatives of the College of Physicians and Surgeons

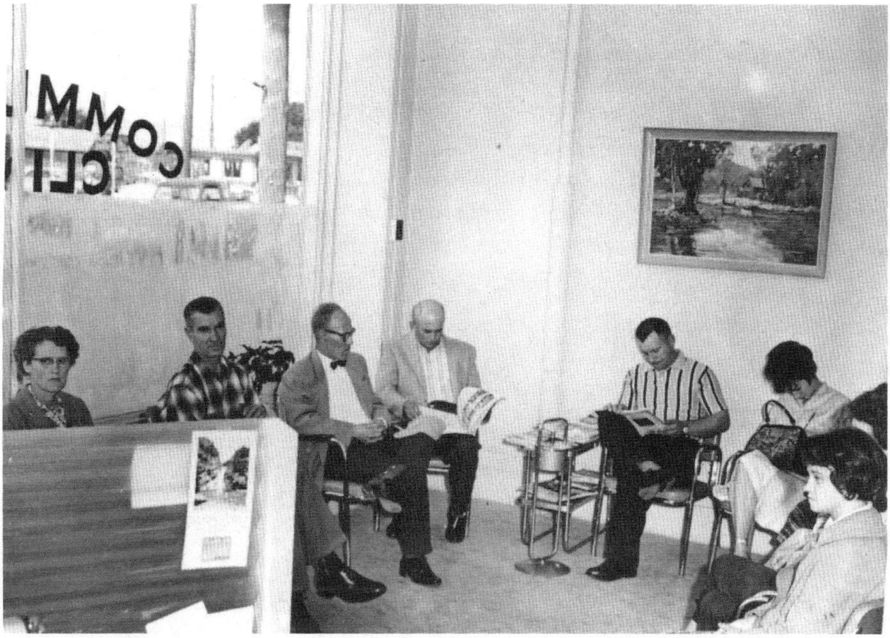

Waiting room, Prince Albert Community Clinic, c. 1963 (Prince Albert Community Clinic, photo #17-PA).

who negotiated with the government in 1962 opposed any provision which might give regulatory powers to the Medical Care Insurance Commission. The College viewed them as steps toward setting up an alternative to itself as the final authority over medical matters in the province.[11]

At the time, neither the news media nor the public paid much attention to these features of the Saskatoon Agreement. Section 14, on the other hand, aroused the attention of clinic doctors and all persons involved in the community associations, for it authorized citizens to "establish premises and invite doctors who wish to enroll for direct payment to rent such premises and set up practice in them." Although not incorporated in the legislation ("Unless abuses arise," the Agreement states, "there is no legislation needed here"), this provision formally acknowledged the legitimacy of community clinics. However, it also limited the role of citizen groups severely: "The role of the citizen group in the provision of insured services must be limited to that of landlord. The only condition which the citizens can properly lay down is that the doctor or doctors in their premises shall be enrolled for direct payment."[12]

The Saskatoon Agreement did make medical services available again, and it did clear the way for the medical care insurance plan to proceed, but community clinic doctors and board members were shocked at the restrictions the Agreement placed on their clinics. The provincial organization which had been established to co-ordinate and service the activities of local groups had already circulated materials throughout the province declaring the long-term objective of the movement to be "high quality medical services through a community operated group practice utilizing payment for certain services provided under the Medical Care Insurance Act." Section 14 of the Saskatoon Agreement threatened to limit the extent to which community clinic organizations could pursue their goals. Could a clinic be "community operated" if the role of the community association was restricted to that of landlord?

Despite these uncertainties, most local association boards continued working to set up their clinics. Some assumed that ways would be found to develop group practice clinics as originally intended; others went ahead with plans simply to establish clinic premises, assuming that they would be given assistance in obtaining doctors to practice in them. All the local associations took it for granted that the Medical Care Plan would be administered in a way that was supportive of community clinics. But as the months went by, people involved in the clinics came to realize how heavily the dice were loaded against them.

An additional concession changed the legislation on the make-up of the Medical Care Insurance Commission. The Saskatoon Agreement required that three additional doctors be added to the Commission, and that these three be approved by the Saskatchewan College of Physicians and Surgeons as well as by the government. This meant, in effect, that the additional members were to represent the interests of the organized medical profession, and that MCIC policies would have to accommodate the desire of the medical establishment that community clinics not develop.

The impact of these concessions was compounded by the organization of the province's medical profession. In Saskatchewan, the College of Physicians and Surgeons and the Saskatchewan Division of the Canadian Medical Association were one and the same. In all other provinces, there were two distinct bodies: a college and a medical association. The College had responsibility for protecting the public interest by licensing doctors, setting standards, and exercising disciplinary powers. The Medical Association, in the other provinces, was limited to protecting the interests of its members, including negotiating economic matters on their behalf. According to a brief presented to the Advisory Planning Committee on Medical Care, "This is surely a rare example of judge, jury, prosecution, and defence rolled into one, and operating in camera."[13] The brief continued: "We believe that the Government of Saskatchewan has been sadly remiss in not bringing this Province abreast of other provinces in this respect." Four years later, the federal Royal Commission on Health Services also recommended that in all provinces the functions of professional self-interest and of public protection be assigned to two separate bodies.[14] In the meantime, the fact that the College represented the economic interest of its members and also exercised licensing and disciplinary powers placed the leaders of the profession in a strong position to influence individual doctors.

A second aspect of the organization of medical practice in Saskatchewan that seriously affected the impact of the concessions had to do with hospital privileges. Saskatchewan doctors are required to seek permission to care for their patients in hospital when hospital care is required. In general it had become almost automatic that, when doctors set up practice in a community, they were accorded the "privilege" of caring for their patients in the local hospital. If questions arose with regard to the suitability or competence of a particular doctor, they were customarily dealt with by the medical staff of the hospital or by a committee of doctors practising in that hospital. Formally, the granting of hospital privileges rested with the hospital board; in practice, hospital boards and administrators were guided by the advice of medical committees. There was no appeal procedure—neither to the health department nor the hospital association, nor even to the College of Physicians and Surgeons. Thus, in situations where a denial of hospital privileges was the result of differing opinion as to how medical care should be organized, the minority view would be suppressed.

Section 11 of the Saskatoon Agreement reads:

> There must be no discrimination against any doctor in whatsoever way he practices. In particular there must be no discrimination against any doctor in the matter of hospital privileges and attachments, referrals from one physician to another, or other professional activities involving assistance and co-operation between physicians. The College endorses this view. It is no wish of the College that there should grow up division between physicians, and it will use its full influence to prevent discrimination in matters of professional practice. Accordingly, the College undertakes that in advising on applications of hospital appointments applicants shall be judged solely on their merits.[15]

It is clear that the parties to the Agreement recognized the need to change discriminatory policies. However, no action was taken, either by legislative amendment or otherwise, to put teeth into this section of the Saskatoon Agreement. Almost 10 months later, the government appointed a commission of inquiry to look into discriminatory practices in the granting of hospital privileges. Dr. W.P. Thompson, chair of the Advisory Planning Committee on Medical Care, summarized its findings: the report of the commission "appears to leave little doubt that the withholding of hospital privileges is being used by the organized medical profession as a weapon in its fight with community clinics and their doctors."[16] The experiences of community clinic doctors makes clear that this discrimination extended not only to applications for hospital privileges, but to all the forms of normal co-operation among doctors as listed in section 11.

The Saskatoon Agreement saved medicare, at least in the short run, but medicare only in the limited sense of an insurance scheme covering mainly doctors' services.[b] It also formally authorized community clinics—in the sense of a citizens' organization providing premises for doctors who were willing to submit their bills to the MCIC—but at the same time it placed serious obstacles in their way. The settlement further involved three amendments to the Medical Care Insurance Act which had implications for community clinics: one deleted provision for an Advisory Council which could have provided an arena for public debate; a second deleted all references to quality of care; a third permitted the medical establishment to appoint three additional members to the Commission.

Almost as important as the legislative changes, however, were the features of the province's medical organization which should have been addressed but were not. No action was taken to separate the licensing body from the economic arm of the medical profession, nor to provide an effective appeal procedure to protect individual doctors from discrimination at the hands of the majority.

[b] Since 1962, the Saskatoon Agreement has often been viewed as restricting the potential of primary health care in Canada by privileging physicians and fee-for-service remuneration: see John Conway, "It's Time for Canada to Finish Medicare's Job," *Journal of Public Health Policy* 10, no. 2 (1989): 157–60.

Notes

1. Community Health Services Association (Saskatchewan), "Provincial Association Brief to the Minister of Public Health" (March 21, 1963).

2. Ibid.

3. Government of Saskatchewan, "Memorandum of Agreement with the College of Physicians and Surgeons of Saskatchewan" ("The Saskatoon Agreement"), (1962).

4. Government of Saskatchewan, Department of Public Health, "Selected Briefs to the Advisory Planning Committee on Medical Care," Vol. 1 (1961).

5. Government of Saskatchewan, "Interim Report of the Advisory Planning Committee on Medical Care" (1961).

6. W.G. Davies moves second reading of Bill 2, "An Act to Amend the Saskatchewan Medical Care Insurance Act, 1961" (Legislative Assembly of Saskatchewan: Debates and Proceedings, Fourth Session, Fourteenth Legislature, August 2, 1962), 5–14.

7. E.A. Tollefson, *Bitter Medicine: The Saskatchewan Medicare Feud* (Saskatoon: Modern Press, 1963), 117.

8. Government of Saskatchewan, "The Saskatchewan Medical Care Insurance Act," Assented to November 17, 1961 in Chapter 1 of the *Statutes of Saskatchewan* (Second Session, 1961).

9. Interdepartmental Committee to Study Medical Care Insurance, "Organized Medicine's Official Position on Health Insurance" (1959), 1–4.

10. Saskatoon Agreement.

11. Badgley and Wolfe, *The Doctors' Strike.*

12. Saskatoon Agreement.

13. Advisory Planning Briefs.

14. *Royal Commission on Health Services, Vol. 1* (Ottawa: Queen's Printer, 1964).

15. Saskatoon Agreement.

16. "Report of the Honourable Mr. Justice Mervyn Woods on Hospital Staff Appointments," Established by Order in Council: 798/63 and 953/63 (Regina: December 11, 1963).

Chapter 5
The Recruiting Problem

Without physicians, the new community clinics could not function. Local clinic associations and the provincial CHSA, therefore, placed the highest priority on recruiting them. Unfortunately, their combined efforts could not tear down the roadblocks set up by government and the organized medical profession.

By November 1962, four months after the signing of the Saskatoon Agreement, 23 doctors were practising in community clinics across Saskatchewan. Nine were Canadians who had joined the clinics when they began. The other 14 were British doctors who had come to serve during the emergency. Some of the latter were committed to the ideal of consumer-sponsored group practice and were resolved to stay; others continued to work in the clinics while they decided whether to return to Britain. Twelve months later, the clinic medical staffs had swelled to 42, but an additional 90 physicians were still required to meet the minimum needs of clinics that were ready to open and to supplement the group practices of those clinics already in operation.

It was late in 1962 that clinic associations realized that Britain would be their chief source of doctors. All Saskatchewan physicians had been invited to apply, but none had responded since the emergency period. Advertising across Canada was limited, as the *Canadian Medical Journal* refused to carry any notices for community clinics; not surprisingly, few applications were received. Outside the country, only graduates of medical schools from the United Kingdom, Ireland, and New Zealand were permitted to register in Saskatchewan without further training. Thus, the large pool of medical professionals south of the border was excluded.

The restriction against American doctors was based not on concerns about their qualifications, but on political pressure from the medical profession and the Saskatchewan government. Had the latter supported the clinic recruitment drive, the College of Physicians and Surgeons might have been forced to remove its restrictions on American doctors. The government might also have insisted on the separation of the College's licensing functions from its association function (as we have seen, in 1962 there was only the College of Physicians and Surgeons; the Saskatchewan Medical Association did not yet exist). With no such support forthcoming, the CHSA and local associations were left to pursue three main recruiting channels: direct contacts in Saskatchewan, advertising (albeit limited) across Canada, and a campaign in Britain.

From the beginning, local associations had been approaching doctors in their own and neighbouring communities. Few of these efforts bore fruit, as it took considerable courage for a Saskatchewan doctor to join a clinic in the face of concerted opposition from his peers.[a] Those who did brought great strength to the clinics, but few dared take the step. Nonetheless, throughout 1963 the clinic movement continued to function in the hope that, as they became better established, many more Saskatchewan doctors would join them.

Although advertising from community clinics was rejected by the *Canadian Medical Journal*, the associations were able to place advertisements regularly in the *Canadian Doctor*, which circulated in all provinces. They also wrote to new graduates of medical schools in Alberta and Manitoba, and sent recruiting posters to all Canadian hospitals that trained interns. They made extensive personal contacts across the country, and advertised in the *British Medical Journal*, which has a large circulation in Canada. During the later months of 1963, a number of inquiries from Canadian doctors—a few of them specialists—trickled in, and correspondence with some continued for months. The result of these efforts in Canada, however, was minimal. It was simply too daunting for most individual physicians to face the censure of the entire medical profession.

By far the most successful recruiting effort was carried out in the United Kingdom. The CHSA arranged with Dr. Terence Gardiner, a respected leader in British medical organizations, to begin a campaign in England in September 1962. Dr. Gardiner had worked in Saskatchewan during the withdrawal of medical services on a one-month contract with the Medical Care Insurance Commission. As he became familiar with the situation, he grew enthusiastic about community clinics and agreed to be the CHSA recruiting representative in the United Kingdom.

Throughout the winter of 1962–63, Gardiner carried on a continuous campaign of advertising and interviewing, and processed over 200 inquiries in Britain. He had to eliminate nearly a quarter of these because they lacked the qualifications to register in Saskatchewan, or were otherwise unsuitable. With the CHSA, he negotiated with about 150 of the remaining applicants. Sometimes that winter it appeared that upwards of 30 qualified physicians were ready to come to Saskatchewan, and many local associations were anticipating their doctors' imminent arrival.[1]

Most of them never came. There were a number of reasons for this. Some were circumstantial: a serious illness in the doctor's family, a personal ailment, better job offers in the United Kingdom. Some doctors, however, encountered unexpected immigration difficulties. Others wrote to medical organizations for information about setting up practice in Saskatchewan, and were strongly discouraged from coming. Still others received letters from Saskatchewan doctors who warned them that they would face great difficulties if they joined a community clinic. A number of the British applicants

[a] Women also practiced medicine in the clinics. Dr. Joan Witney-Moore was the first doctor to join the Saskatoon Community Clinic in 1962, and Dr. Margaret Mahood, a psychiatrist, joined this same year: see Dennis Gruending, *The First Ten Years* (Saskatoon: Community Health Services Association (Saskatoon) Ltd., 1973) and, for the role of female physicians in the Regina clinic, Margaret Hughes, *A Biography: The Community Health Center Regina* (Regina: Community Health Services Association (Regina) Ltd., 1977), 31. A recent survey of doctors in Québec, a jurisdiction that features both fee-for-service doctors and a network of community health centres with salaried doctors found that women are twice as likely as men to work under salary: see André-Pierre Contandriopoulos et Marc-André Fournier, *Féminisation de la profession médicale et transformation de la pratique au Québec* (Montréal: Groupe de recherche interdisciplinaire en santé, Faculté de médecine, Université de Montréal, 2007).

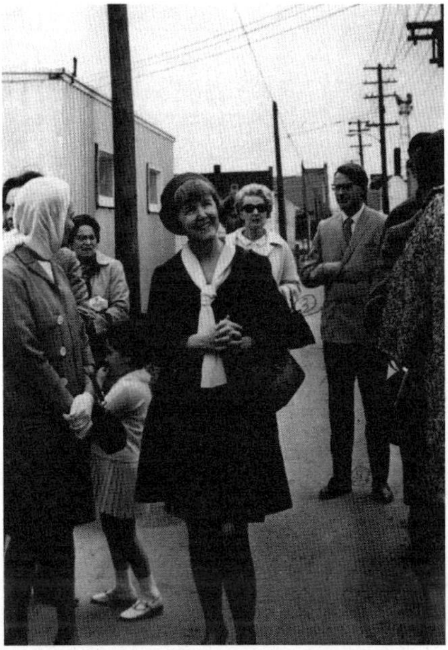

Dr. Margaret Mahood (centre) at sod-turning ceremony for new community clinic building in Saskatoon (Saskatoon Community Clinic, photo # 4-SK).

were personally approached by representatives of Saskatchewan groups opposed to the medical care plan.[2]

Articles in medical journals and British newspapers painted a biased picture of the Saskatchewan medical plan. Even the news of the Woods Commission hearings into discrimination in regard to hospital privileges (May–June 1963) had an adverse effect. Dr. Gardiner noted that media reports of the Commission caused several recruits to hesitate or withdraw. Because the Woods Commission was investigating the cases of doctors from the United Kingdom, potential recruits inferred that Saskatchewan people were hostile to British doctors.

Inevitably, the number of doctors who actually arrived by the summer of 1963 was much lower than the CHSA had anticipated. Local associations, some with premises ready and standing idle, were bitterly disappointed. Many community clinic supporters lacked access to medical care. Some had no doctor at all.

The provincial board of the Community Health Services Associations decided that a special recruiting effort was needed during the summer of 1963. Dr. Gardiner asked the CHSA to send a team from Saskatchewan to help make a concerted drive for recruits. The CHSA selected Dr. Samuel Wolfe and the author, Stan Rands, to spend two weeks with Dr. Gardiner in Britain at the end of the summer. Sam Wolfe was Medical Consultant to the provincial CHSA, as well as Medical Director of the Saskatoon Community Clinic. I was the Director of the CHSA.

Dr. Gardiner was well prepared. He had advertised extensively, and interviewed many new applicants as well as renewing contacts with doctors who had been hesitating. Over the course of two weeks we interviewed about 45 doctors. Of these, Dr. Gardiner recommended 30 as being both highly skilled and interested in joining community clinics. We interviewed most of the applicants, not individually but in groups, for two days each. This allowed us to give them a more complete picture both of Saskatchewan and of community clinics. It also allowed us to answer many of their questions and weed out those recruits who would likely be neither comfortable nor successful working in the conditions doctors encountered at that time in Saskatchewan.

It is a big step for anyone to pull up roots and move to a completely new setting, especially in the midst of controversy. Inevitably, our intensive recruiting effort was not as fruitful as we had hoped. It took months for some recruits to wind up their affairs in Britain, some accepted other job offers, and, as before, some were contacted by the opposition and persuaded not to come.

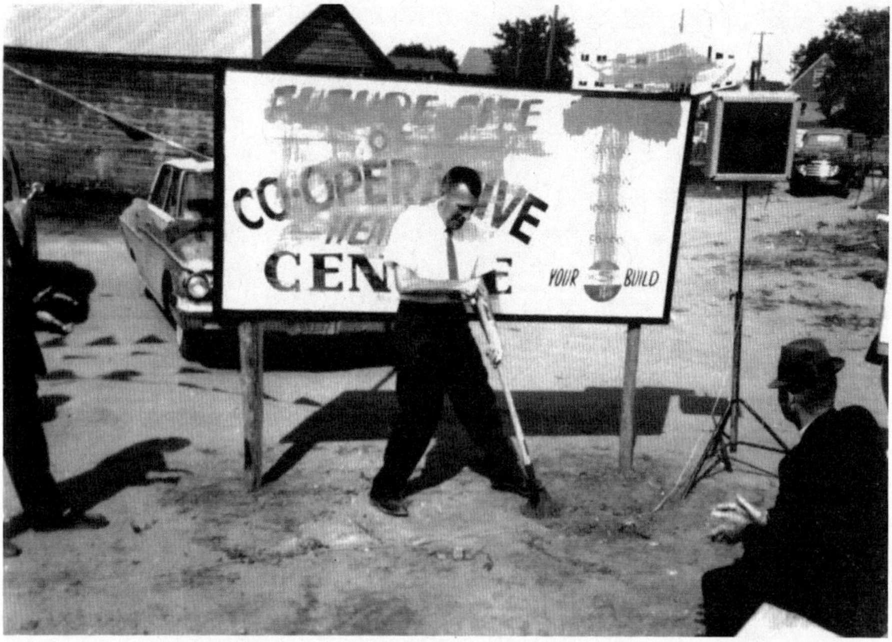

Dr. Hjertaas opening the new Co-operative Health Centre in Prince Albert, in front of a sign that was defaced the night before (Prince Albert Community Clinic, photo #7-PA).

That we did succeed in recruiting 30 doctors, most of whom came across an ocean and half a continent to a forbidding landscape amid daunting stigma and heavy personal, financial, and political pressure, was a major accomplishment. It was an accomplishment that reflected the dedication of community members who risked both their savings to build clinics, and their personal health while they waited for doctors to arrive. It also reflected a courageous commitment on the part of doctors who cared enough about health care to accept the risks of working in community clinics under almost siege conditions.

It was direct interference from the medical profession and lack of support from the provincial government that took the heaviest toll on recruiting efforts. If the medical profession and the Keep Our Doctors committees had not intimidated physicians in Saskatchewan and across Canada, many more would certainly have accepted work in community clinics. If the provincial government had taken a more active role in recruiting, facilitating immigration, and certifying doctors—that is, if it had challenged the CMA—the recruitment could have been far more effective. Without government support, individual community associations were left with voluntary donations and limited political expertise to overcome the massed opposition of the entire medical profession.

Certainly, some communities were divided. Some were suspicious of foreign doctors, and at least one rejected a recruit because of his race. But these internal stresses were minor compared to the massive external pressures brought to bear against the community clinics. As Sam Wolfe pointed out, Saskatchewan communities had over

40 years' experience with co-operative medicine, and the concept of consumer-sponsored comprehensive group practice had been thought out and welcomed long before the medicare crisis.[3]

In the absence of overt support from the government, the effort to recruit doctors was impressive. But it was not enough.

Notes

1. Rose Potvin (ed.), *Passion and Conviction: The Letters of Graham Spry* (Regina: Canadian Plains Research Center, 1992).

2. Stan Rands interviews.

3. Robin F. Badgley and Samuel Wolfe, *The Doctors' Strike: Medical Care and Conflict in Saskatchewan* (Toronto: MacMillan of Canada, 1976).

Chapter 6
The Financial Picture: High Expectations, Low Income

The financial problems encountered by community clinics during their first few years of operation both impaired efforts to establish new clinics and severely hampered operations in those clinics that already existed. Community health associations had expected support from the Medical Care Insurance Commission; they saw co-operative clinics as an extension of the medicare plan, which they had strongly supported. Also, CCF-NDP officials had actively endorsed the clinic organizing campaign during the doctors' withdrawal of services. Prominent New Democrats from as far away as Ontario visited rural communities in Saskatchewan to encourage local committees. And the well-publicized "air-lift" of British doctors carried out by the MCIC to provide medical services in places where doctors had closed their offices led associations to believe that the Commission would help them find doctors who were willing to practice under medicare.

There were further grounds for optimism after the signing of the Saskatoon Agreement on July 23. Clinic organizing groups in about 20 communities sent representatives to a series of province-wide meetings to pool their information and experience. They formed a provincial committee to co-ordinate joint actions, incorporating it as the Community Health Services (Saskatchewan) Association. On August 20, the executive of the provincial association met with Premier Lloyd to discuss the progress and prospects of the Community Health Associations.

Tommy Shoyama,[a] then Chairman of the Economic Advisory and Planning Board and one of five officials who had worked with Lord Taylor to produce the Saskatoon Agreement, accompanied the Premier to the meeting and took detailed notes. He sent a copy of his record of the meeting to the executive of the provincial CHSA. They clearly implied that the government wanted the clinics to succeed. Premier Lloyd indicated that the government would have to consider what help to the citizen groups would be appropriate in view of the uneasy relations with the medical profession and "the reported concern and apprehension on the part of the organized profession over

[a] T.K. Shoyama (1916–2006) joined the provincial government as a research economist in 1946. Four years later, he became secretary to the Economic Advisory and Planning Board (EAPB) and Douglas's closest policy advisor. When Douglas left the premiership in November 1961 to become leader of the national New Democratic Party, Shoyama took a leave of absence to act as an advisor. He returned to the provincial government as head of the EAPB shortly after Douglas's defeat in Regina in the federal election of June 1962 in large part due to the bitterness of the medicare struggle and the imminent doctors' strike. In 1964, after the Lloyd government's defeat, Shoyama left Saskatchewan for Ottawa where he would eventually become Deputy Minister of Finance. See Houston and Waiser, *Tommy's Team*, 163–68.

the emergence of the community clinics." At the same time the Premier suggested that the clinics could be viewed as contributing to the medical insurance program in three specific ways:

> 1. facilitating the increase in the number of physicians enrolled for direct payment;
>
> 2. emphasizing quality of care and health education of citizens;
>
> 3. unifying community groups for co-operative action in support of the insurance program.

Shoyama's notes continued:

> There were obvious precedents for government assistance to such citizens groups, either because of their co-operative structure and organization, or because of their promotion of better health for individuals and communities.[1]

Premier Lloyd supported government assistance to the CHSA groups both generally and specifically. He agreed that the CHSA could expect help from Saskatchewan House, London, in recruiting British doctors. He further agreed "that the discussions [of CHSA] with the Commission [MCIC] should include a request that the Commission contribute to the costs of interviewing British doctors and that some arrangements be worked out concerning the advance of travel and settlement costs as an aid to recruitment." He also felt it would be appropriate for the CHSA to discuss physician recruitment with the Medical Care Insurance Commission.

Of paramount importance to CHSA representatives was the matter of salaries. The executive stressed that the survival of community clinics depended on the MCIC continuing the policy it had implemented during the doctors' withdrawal of services, namely, paying physicians directly in accordance with a salary schedule based on training and experience. The record of the meeting suggests that the Premier and/or his lieutenant were sympathetic to the urging of the CHSA that salaries paid by the MCIC be extended to include those community clinic doctors who desired it.

The August meeting between the Premier and the CHSA executive would have been an appropriate time to issue a warning if the government had seen community clinics as a threat to the medicare plan or to the political future of the government. In the absence of such a warning, the provincial executive of the CHSA felt confident in encouraging local associations to continue their efforts to establish or maintain their clinics.

On October 1, 1962, the Medical Care Insurance Commission sent the provincial CHSA a copy of Minute 304 in response to a CHSA request for clarification of MCIC policy:

> 304. The Commission considered a proposal from the Provincial Association of Community Health Services Associations respecting the conditions under which the Commission will authorize fixed payment contracts with physicians practising in association with member groups.
>
> The Commission agreed that it would enter into contracts with suitable physicians on the following basis: a) that the request for fixed

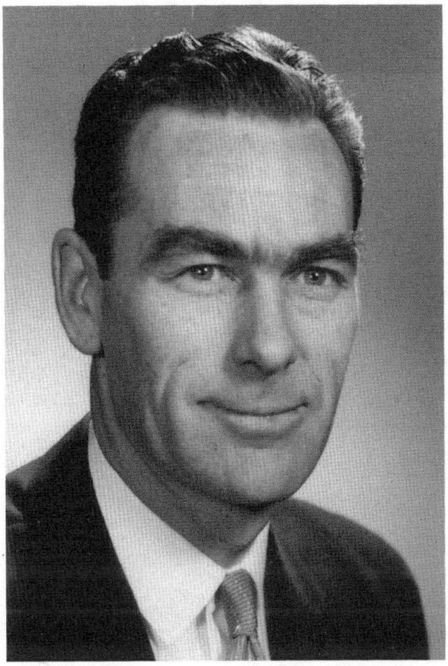

Don Tansley, Chair of the Medical Care Insurance Commission, 1961–64 (SAB R-10698).

payment remuneration originate with the physician; b) that, in any association, one physician contract be allotted for each 350 certified family memberships.

Further conditions specified in the minute were that the doctor report services "in a manner satisfactory to the Commission," that the doctor's service load be reviewed periodically, and that "continuing study be given to the basis of allotment and the methods of evaluation."[2]

The provincial CHSA executive felt that the quota of 350 families was too high and the salary scales offered by MCIC too low, but that the ruling "constitutes definite progress." The executive felt that part of the Commission's minute provided the mechanics for revising the 350 figure, for the government had also agreed, following the August 20 meeting, to urge the MCIC to raise the salary scales offered to doctors. Consequently, the provincial CHSA office sent copies of Minute 304 to all its locals, urging them to bring their memberships up to 350 or, in communities desiring two doctors, to 700. It also advised associations that in the light of the new MCIC ruling, the CHSA recruiting representative in Britain would recruit doctors for fixed payment contracts.

There were still more than 100 municipal doctor plans in Saskatchewan in January 1962, so salary or contract payment was not uncommon. Officially, the Medical Care Insurance Commission was willing to continue such arrangements, as indicated in its 1962 Annual Report: "Individual physicians who wished might elect to be paid on a fixed payment basis."[3]

Don Tansley, MCIC chairperson, attended the November Annual Meeting of the Saskatchewan CHSA and outlined Commission policy on salaries for doctors. The Commission was prepared, he said, to offer a fixed salary to a community clinic doctor once the local association had signed up 350 members. Salaries based on training, experience, and the local situation—would range from $12,000 to $40,000 gross. Mr. Tansley made it clear that the CHSA recruiting officer in the United Kingdom could make no advance commitment to any British physician because the Commission would make the final decision on each contract.[4]

A year later, the report of the provincial CHSA board of directors to the Second Annual Meeting stated:

It has proven impossible for any of our community clinic doctors to obtain a satisfactory fixed-payment contract with the Medical Care Insurance Commission, as had been expected at the time of last year's convention. All the community clinic doctors bill the Medical Care Insurance Commission directly on a fee-for-service basis.[5]

In March 1963, the CHSA presented a brief to the provincial cabinet outlining the progress and problems of the community clinics, and making specific requests. The brief emphasized the stultifying effects of MCIC policy and practice:

> Fixed-payment contracts at an adequate level would be a substantial help in recruiting doctors for community clinics. Dr. Terence Gardiner advises us that some of the best specialists have withdrawn their applications when they have learned that they cannot get fixed-payment contracts. These men have always worked on salary and they abhor the idea of practising on a fee per item of service. Other doctors have come on the basis of guaranteed minimum incomes and have been distressed to discover the cumbersome financial and contractual arrangements forced upon the clinics by the need to arrange guaranteed minimum incomes within the fee-for-service system.
>
> Fixed-payment contracts would attract more doctors of the kind the clinics need—those who are interested in quality of service rather than volume of income.[6]

The brief also explained the disastrous results of the MCIC's failure to follow through on the 350-family formula, and it challenged the actions of the Commission as being inconsistent with its own terms of reference in the Saskatoon Agreement and the Medical Care Insurance Act.

Even those clinics that managed to start up and stay open encountered serious problems with the government and the medical establishment. Physicians who had come from Britain and from other provinces to provide medical services during the boycott did so on a fixed-payment contract—in effect, a salary. They expected that method to continue. The Community Health Services Associations made the same assumption, and financial planning was done on that basis. With doctors on a fixed salary, a reasonable rent—the only source of funding for ongoing operating costs—could be easily calculated.

When the Commission finally ruled, early in 1963, that payments to community clinic doctors must be on a fee-for-service basis, it was a severe blow. To compound the burden, the arrangement was made retroactive to July 1962. Community clinic staff were thus forced to go back over more than six months of patient charts, transferring to MCIC claim cards each service that had been rendered by a clinic doctor. As the business manager of one of these "successful" clinics recalls, this put a tremendous strain on the support staff:

> A lot of night work had to be done to catch up on this backlog. For part of the period we had to go through the same grind for laboratory services. These were some of the enormous obstacles which prevented us getting ahead with creative planning. It was a strain on the medical director, too, as he was trying to integrate British doctors who were not familiar with fee-for-service. It was a strain on the lay board as well because of the tremendous financial implications. There were also the legal problems. A great deal of time and money went into trying to straighten out the legal relationships of the association with the doctors and with the government. It would have made an enormous difference if the government had given support.[7]

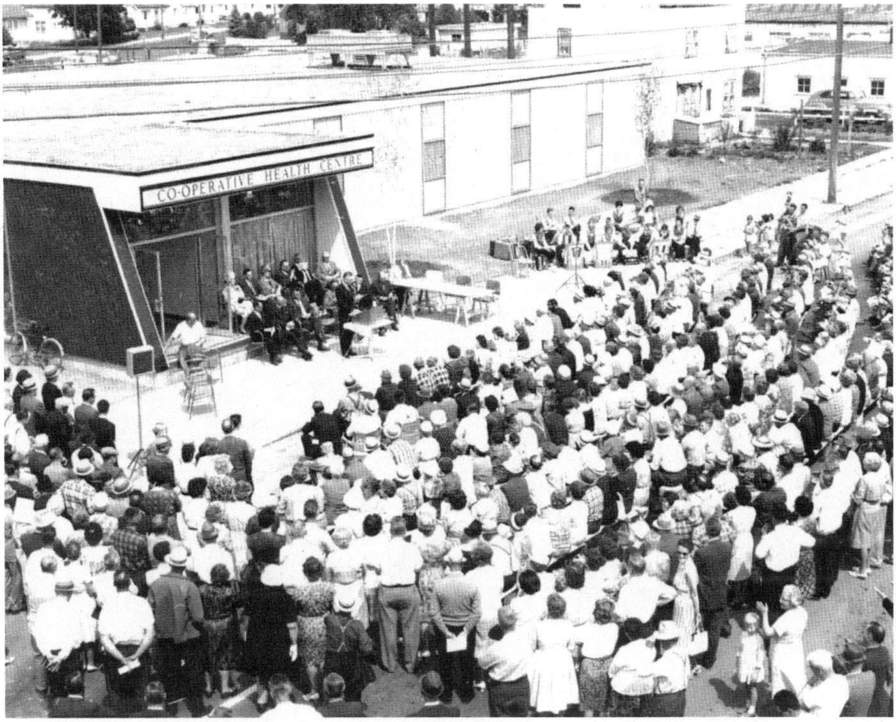

Grand opening of the new Prince Albert Co-operative Health Centre in 1964 (Prince Albert Community Clinic, photo #13-PA).

Raising money for buildings and equipment was not a major problem in most areas. It was operating expenses that threatened to close the clinics. And that would not have been a problem if they had immediately begun practising medicine. The caseload would have built up quickly, as the clinics had a ready-made clientele of members and other citizens who wanted medical services paid for directly by the MCIC. As the Eston Association reported at the time, "There are enough patients waiting for our two doctors to arrive to keep them busy for the next eight months."

Unfortunately, recruiting obstructions caused a number of associations to pay out money for building maintenance for months without any income. As well, difficulties in obtaining hospital privileges for community clinic physicians kept a large proportion of potential users from attending the clinics. It also made it necessary for clinic doctors to refer elsewhere all but the low-fee procedures. These and other factors kept medical income at such a low level that associations had to underwrite all operating expenses and, in most cases, subsidize their doctors' incomes.

Members of all local health associations had contributed money cheerfully in the belief that their objectives were worthwhile. But in several locations the prospects of the financial picture improving were so distant that members hesitated to go deeper into debt. By the end of 1963, three clinics in the province were seriously considering closing down, and there was a danger of despair spreading to other centres—although, in general, morale was still high in most associations. There were few real problems that some tangible assistance could not have overcome.

Notes

1. Stan Rands, personal notes.
2. MCIC, Minute 304, October 1962.
3. MCIC, *Annual Report*, 1962.
4. CHSA, Annual Meeting, November 1962.
5. CHSA, Annual Meeting, November 1963.
6. CHSA, Brief to Provincial Cabinet, March 1963.
7. Stan Rands, interview with Michael Kalmakoff.

Chapter 7
Kindersley: A Case Study in Policy Failure

In the effort to launch a clinic in Kindersley we see reflected many of the experiences of Community Health Associations across Saskatchewan. Every community has its unique features, but Kindersley is fairly typical in terms of effort expended, problems encountered, and eventual outcome. The town and surrounding area also are fairly representative in terms of population profile, social and economic activity, and history.

In 1962, the town and its trading area had a combined population of around 6,500. Situated in wheat-growing country near one of the oil and gas fields that hug the Saskatchewan-Alberta border, it is approximately 200 kilometres from Saskatoon and 400 kilometres from Calgary. The CCF had been returned in each election from 1944 through to the medicare election of 1960, with the runner-up a Liberal in all but one instance.

During June 1962, the people of Kindersley, like their fellow citizens across the province, speculated about the Medical Care Insurance Plan and the threatened boycott of the plan by Saskatchewan physicians. But it was not until the plan actually went into effect on July 1 that people realized the boycott was also going into effect. Even then, many people could not believe that their doctors had actually withdrawn their services. There was a feeling among some residents, however, that something had to be done. An informal gathering took place in a Kindersley home the following afternoon.

This original group of 12 people began organizing to deal with the emergency, forming a Community Health Services Association and putting in place the first tentative plans for a clinic. Even after the Saskatoon Agreement was signed on July 23, they continued organizing, for they were concerned about what the Agreement implied. A public meeting, in fact, was held the next day, July 24. Attendance was reported at well over 500, and it was clear that the majority wanted the medicare plan to succeed.

When the public meeting ended, the local CHSA met and elected a permanent board of directors. At this meeting a family membership fee was set at $5, with $1 of that payable to the provincial organization; this was indicative of the Kindersley Association's awareness of the need for co-ordinated action across the province. By the end of July, 133 families had joined the local Association and $133 had been sent to the provincial Association.

Over the next two months the Kindersley CHSA directors worked exhaustively; only two doctors had returned after the boycott and, aside from the serious shortage of medical services this represented, the two doctors that did return refused to send their bills to the Medical Care Insurance Commission. Patients were thus required to pay their doctor directly and eventually be reimbursed by the MCIC. CHSA members felt that they would not receive the full benefits of medicare until they had the opportunity to choose a doctor who was practising under the plan. The CHSA Board therefore concentrated on finding two doctors who would be willing to rent premises from the Association and send their bills to the Medical Care Insurance Commission.

Accordingly, they sent $500 to the provincial Association to help it recruit doctors, and they themselves began corresponding with a doctor in Hong Kong who, they had been told, was interested in coming to Canada. They took options on a building to use temporarily as a clinic, and purchased two lots for a permanent clinic in the future. They purchased $500 worth of clinical equipment so there would be no delay should doctors arrive on short notice. Although it was estimated that nearly half of the approximately 1,400 families in the area supported plans for the clinic, the Board decided to hold back on an all-out drive for members until doctors were in sight. Even so, family memberships had grown to 300 by the end of November.

In view of the limitations placed on clinics and local Health Associations by the Saskatoon Agreement, and because of the medical establishment's overt hostility to community clinics, the CHSA Board in Kindersley had to exercise extreme caution in observing the letter of the law. It frequently sought advice from both the legal consultant and the medical advisor to the provincial CHSA. Model contracts worked out by these provincial consultants precariously balanced the Saskatoon Agreement's prohibition against Associations taking any role but landlord with their legitimate desire to become more actively involved. The Kindersley Association registered under the Mutual Medical and Hospital Benefits Associations Act, which gave it the right to make agreements with doctors to provide services.

In late November 1962, the provincial CHSA held its first annual convention in Saskatoon. This gave all the local Associations an opportunity to meet, discuss their mutual and individual problems, and chart a course for the future. The Kindersley Association sent twelve delegates, and during the two days of discussions they urged the CHSA to concentrate its energies on securing doctors to practise in community clinics. The Kindersley delegates found it hard to believe that the Medical Care Insurance Commission, which had actively recruited temporary doctors from Britain and elsewhere during the boycott, would not help in recruiting doctors for communities such as theirs. Officers of the provincial Association, who had raised the matter more than once with MCIC officials, had the difficult task of explaining a policy with which they themselves were in strong disagreement. The Kindersley delegates returned home with the political support of the provincial Association, but they were no closer to a solution to their basic predicament.

The Kindersley Association felt that they were being let down. They had developed an organization that enjoyed strong support from the town and surrounding area. They had elected a representative, responsible, and hard-working Board. They had mastered the intricate legalities of a situation that was entirely new to all of them. They had made all the necessary preparations to put a clinic in operation on short notice once a couple of doctors were available. But neither they nor the provincial Association could recruit doctors without government support.

This feeling of betrayal dominated the meeting of the Kindersley Board on December 8, 1962, when the convention delegates made their report. Feelings ran high, and the discussion was unusually heated. Some felt the MCIC was pushing the Association into the position of doing battle, not with the Keep Our Doctors committees or the medical profession, but with the very government which had brought in medicare. Delegates were particularly irked at the reasons they had been given for the MCIC's inability to help areas like Kindersley obtain doctors; i.e., the Medical Care Insurance Commission was permitted to supply doctors only to "under-doctored" areas, and "under-doctored" had been interpreted to mean *no* doctors.

The Kindersley Association sent a strongly worded letter to the MCIC, pointing out that the area had fewer doctors than it needed for good service and no doctor at all operating under Category 1 of the Act, which meant, in effect, that patients had no freedom of choice as to the kind of doctor they might go to. The term "under-doctored," the letter went on, had been compared at the Board meeting with terms such as "underfed" and "undereducated," and it was felt that only educated fools could get away with the idea that "under-doctored" could mean having no doctor at all. The letter concluded with a request for assistance in getting a doctor or doctors who would bill the Commission directly and give those of the Kindersley area who wished it an opportunity to exercise their freedom of choice in going to a doctor.[1]

The Kindersley Board's plea to the MCIC did not bring about a change of policy, but they continued to co-operate with the provincial Association's recruiting efforts and to follow up on leads of their own. Before the end of the year, they began to negotiate with a doctor from a neighbouring town who had expressed an interest in practising in Kindersley. In July 1963, the physician finally began renting the Kindersley clinic building. Then, because of pressure from other doctors, the newcomer became increasingly unwilling to send bills directly to the MCIC or to deal with the Association as a tenant.

Because many other local Associations were desperate for doctors, the provincial Association sent a recruiting team to the United Kingdom in August 1963. Kindersley provided detailed information to the provincial officers concerning the conditions in the town and area, the type of doctors they most wanted, and those who would most likely be at home there. Using this information and a positive assessment of the support available for a community clinic doctor in Kindersley, the recruiters selected a certain Dr. Jones, one of the several dozen British doctors who had been interviewed in London.

Two CHSA representatives from Saskatchewan, Dr. Sam Wolfe and I, as well as our UK representative, Dr. Terence Gardiner, spent a good deal of time with Dr. Jones. He heard our presentation on the Saskatchewan situation, and he spoke with the three of us, individually and together. We answered all his questions about Kindersley, the medicare plan, financial arrangements, procedures for getting settled into practice, and the climate. Naturally, we informed him of the negative aspects of the situation as well, but at the end of our lengthy sessions he gave us the definite impression that he was making the decision to come. Mrs. Jones, who had also taken part in the conversations, seemed to like the idea of Kindersley and thought she would fit well into the community life. The couple promised us a final decision quickly and indicated that, if their answer was positive, they could come within six weeks.

It was a pleasure to be able to convey to the Kindersley people the prospect of having a doctor of such excellent background so quickly. We assumed that, once one physician joined the clinic, it would be easier to find a second. The Kindersley Association reacted with a flurry of excitement. The Board began a push toward building a clinic that would be more appropriate for two doctors, and expected to have a new building by January 1964 at the latest.

A few weeks later, Dr. Jones wrote that he had decided not to come "for the present." It was painful for the provincial office to have to pass this word to Kindersley. They were of course anxious to hear why the doctor had refused, since his reasons affected their decision about whether to continue the effort to establish a community clinic. If Dr. Jones' decision was based on purely personal factors, they would continue searching for doctors. But if he had been dissuaded by pressure from the College of Physicians and Surgeons, other applicants for community clinic positions would face the same situation. The continued overt hostility of organized medicine to the community clinics, the number of applicants who had been frightened away, and the others who had found themselves isolated and persecuted by their colleagues meant that the provincial Association could offer little hope to the people of Kindersley.

But still the Kindersley Association did not give up. Shortly after the disappointment about Dr. Jones, three representatives from Kindersley came to Regina. I accompanied them to a discussion with the Chairperson and the Medical Director of the Medical Care Insurance Commission. They showed their sketch plan for a clinic building to house three doctors and supplementary services, and asked for comments on the suitability of these plans for the Kindersley district. A review of the number of doctors practising in the area surrounding Kindersley showed clearly that many residents were having to travel considerable distances to be served by a doctor who would send bills directly to the MCIC. The MCIC made useful suggestions concerning the building plans, and provided information on policy related to physiotherapy and laboratory services. But on the most crucial issue, the meeting produced nothing new. MCIC officials saw no way of defining "under-doctored" or "over-doctored" except in terms of the income a doctor would make on a fee-for-service basis, and consequently saw no way to help the local Association obtain doctors.

Members of the Kindersley Association, along with several other local Associations, asked the provincial Association to publicly correct misleading statements made by politicians and hostile doctors, and to expose the harassment faced by community clinic doctors. But the provincial officers, on the advice of doctors working in community clinics, were cautious. One reply to Kindersley read:

> We do not think that anyone from CHSA can make a public statement on this matter without causing difficulty for some of the community clinic doctors. However, it is quite possible that there are people not directly involved with the CHSA who would want to make a public comment. It is a sad commentary that citizens must voluntarily restrict their right to free speech because of the power of a professional pressure group, but that seems to be the situation we are still in.[2]

The doctors practising in community clinics during the 1960s were, in effect, hostages of the College of Physicians and Surgeons. Public statements by the CHSA could be, and sometimes were, used as a basis for disciplinary action against clinic doctors. Disciplinary sanctions were a constant threat not only to clinic doctors, but to the heads of the Associations as well: if clinic doctors were to lose their licenses or be suspended, the clinics themselves could be destroyed.

The Kindersley Association had shown great strength from the beginning. It had able leadership and a broad base of support throughout the district. Many of the members would have liked to carry the fight into the public arena. But few things are more damaging to morale than to be ready for a battle in which you know you are right, but to have your hands tied behind your back.

In the summer of 1965, after two years of frustration, a special membership meeting decided not to begin construction of a clinic in Kindersley, even though $26,000 in loan capital had been secured. The decision was not to give up, but to postpone further investment until doctors became available. Years later, a founding member of the Kindersley Community Health Services Association confided, "We had the basis for a whole new and constructive approach to the delivery of health care, but the government let us down completely."[3]

Many CHSA members were the children and grandchildren of the original settlers who had opened up the area. These were the people who had built the Wheat Pool, local co-operatives, and the credit unions, people who had established the early farm organizations, and eventually the Co-operative Commonwealth Federation (CCF). It was natural for these people to turn to a health co-operative, a community clinic, as a means of defending medicare and getting its full benefits. They saw a clinic owned by the people as a means of escaping the autocratic dominance of medical care in an area served by one establishment doctor.

The CCF had won the Kindersley constituency in five consecutive elections since 1944. In 1964, they lost it.

Notes

1. Stan Rands, private papers, 1962.
2. Ibid.
3. Ibid.

Chapter 8
Trouble With Hospital Privileges

At a press conference on May 11, 1963, Dr. Samuel Wolfe, speaking for community clinic doctors, objected to the apparent attempts of organized medicine not only to keep doctors from joining the clinics but to drive out those doctors who were already working in them. The President of the Saskatchewan College of Physicians and Surgeons, Dr. Harry Portnuff, rejoined that he was surprised that Dr. Wolfe was not more cognizant of the Saskatoon Agreement and of regulations under the Hospital Standards Act. The College, he said, had "nothing whatever to do with applications for staff appointments."[1]

Two weeks later, Dr. George Peacock, Registrar of the College, journeyed with three other doctors to Estevan to take part in a meeting of the Joint Medical and Hospital Standards Committee. Their presence had been requested by Sister Superior Mary Priscilla, administrator of Saint Joseph's Hospital, to review the situation with regard to the application of Dr. P.J. Murphy for hospital privileges. The action of the College in sending its representatives 460 kilometres to attend a meeting that was concerned with specific aspects of an application for hospital privileges is difficult to reconcile with the statement made by the President of the College just two weeks earlier. The inconsistency is underlined by the Registrar's public admission that the applications of Dr. Murphy and a second community clinic doctor were discussed by the Council of the College on March 31 and May 5, and that an Estevan doctor who opposed the clinic there had attended the May 5 meeting to receive the recommendations of the College concerning the applications.

"More community clinic doctors," wrote Samuel Wolfe in the CMA *Journal* of August 1, 1964, "have experienced difficulties in obtaining hospital privileges than all other doctors combined in the history of the province of Saskatchewan." Dr. Wolfe might have used his own case as an example. He had been practising medicine in Saskatchewan for 12 years when he joined the Saskatoon Community Clinic in July 1962. He had been a professor on the Faculty of Medicine at the University of Saskatchewan. He had been appointed by the Saskatchewan Government to the Medical Care Insurance Commission. Yet more than a year after he entered community clinic practice, Saskatoon City Hospital had admitted him only to the probationary medical staff, with limited privileges.

Dr. Wolfe was by no means alone.

The sudden rash of problems having to do with hospital privileges in communities that were operating clinics led CHSA spokespersons to suggest that a campaign against community clinic doctors was being encouraged, if not orchestrated, by the medical establishment through its provincial body, the College of Physicians and Surgeons. This suggestion was vigorously denied by the College. In addition to Dr. Portnuff's statement quoted above, a further statement on June 4, and similar denials by the College Registrar, a statement on behalf of the Saskatchewan Division of the Canadian Medical Association was made by Dr. M.A. Baltzan in the May 18 edition of the Saskatoon *StarPhoenix*. "The Saskatchewan College of Physicians and Surgeons," he wrote, "plays no part in either rejecting or approving any application from one of its members to a hospital." Yet during this same period the Woods Commission[a] on Hospital Staff Appointments produced evidence of the frequent and intimate involvement of the College in individual cases of application for hospital privileges. It was found, for instance, that the medical staff of Saint Joseph's Hospital in Estevan had approached the College for guidance not only on the general question of hospital privileges but with regard to the applications of particular doctors. Concerning the application of Dr. N. Samuels, the Commission reported:

> The application was found to be in order, but no recommendation for its acceptance was made. Instead, the medical staff decided to seek advice and guidance on the whole question of hospital privileges, and to present all pertinent details concerning the application of Dr. Samuels at the next Council meeting of the College of Physicians and Surgeons.
>
> A special meeting of the Executive Committee of the medical staff was held on April 18 for the purpose of considering the special report of the College of Physicians and Surgeons on the question of approving staff-membership for Dr. Samuels.[2]

The hospital privileges controversy was particularly serious for community clinic supporters in rural areas and small towns. Many of these communities had been deeply split over the medicare issue, especially during the withdrawal of doctors' services in July 1962. In most situations, local doctors had led the fight against the plan, whereas many of their patients, rural and small town people, had strongly supported it. When the plan went into operation these people wanted their bills sent to the Medical Care Insurance Commission, for that was the only way they could receive the full benefits of the plan. Hence, they had formed community health services associations and tried to obtain doctors who were willing to bill the MCIC. Now these citizens received an unexpected jolt: their physicians were not being allowed into their local hospitals.

This was a serious issue for anyone, but especially for the elderly, the chronically ill, and families with young children. Who could tell when an illness or an injury might require hospitalization? Denying hospital privileges to community clinic doctors placed people under enormous pressure to give up on the clinic and return to the physicians who had been practising in the community before the crisis—doctors who had opposed

[a] On the personnel, mandate, and outcome of the Royal Commission on Hospital Privileges (known as the Woods Commission because of its chair, Justice Mervyn Woods of the Saskatchewan Court of Appeal), see Roy Romanow, "My Experience in the Medicare Battle and the Woods Commission," *Canadian Bulletin of Medical History* 26, no. 2 (2009): 538–41. Romanow served as assistant secretary to Ed Wahn, the Commission's secretary.

medicare and closed their offices on July 1, 1962. A number of families succumbed, but more often they held out, month after month, in some cases for years.

But the price was high. As one pioneer farmer remarked in the fall of 1962, "I struggled for years to get a hospital in our town and now, 20 years later, I have to drive 50 miles to a hospital because my doctor is not allowed into our own hospital."[3] On the other hand, this awareness of history helped community clinic supporters push forward, despite the obstacles and the hazards.

Saskatchewan's rural people created their own hospitals, the earliest ones erected by co-operative action. People would recognize a need, organize themselves to plan and make decisions, then pool their resources to construct and equip a building in which doctors could provide services for the whole community. From the beginning, Saskatchewan hospitals have been public institutions. Even those hospitals that were owned and controlled by religious orders made services available to the entire community.

Control of hospitals other than those owned by religious orders has traditionally rested with local government bodies: town or city councils, villages, rural municipalities. Hospital boards are appointed by local government bodies and are subject to policies determined by them. Over the decades, tax support has come increasingly from the provincial government, and the federal government has come to shoulder a large part of the cost of hospital construction. Increased funding by senior governments has resulted in greater provincial and federal influence on overall policy, but the responsibility for day-to-day operation has continued to rest with the local government bodies through the hospital boards appointed by them.

Thus, Saskatchewan hospitals are public institutions controlled by bodies that are ultimately responsible to the people. Since all patients have a right to use these institutions, qualified physicians should have equal opportunity to use them also. This has been the assumption historically, but it has not led to an absence of standards. On the contrary, provincial legislation and hospital by-laws have developed over the years to provide safeguards for patients.

Generally speaking, a doctor who was registered with the Saskatchewan College of Physicians and Surgeons and settling into a practice in a town or rural area received hospital privileges almost automatically. In city hospitals the situation was a bit more complex, for general practitioners and specialists were accorded privileges appropriate to their training and experience. Still, it was rare for a qualified physician to be refused hospital privileges.

The position of organized medicine on the issue was clear and definite before 1962. Nationally and provincially, the position of the profession was that hospitals should be "open." In 1957, this position was succinctly expressed by Dr. Morley A.R. Young, then President of the Canadian Medical Association: "Every medical practitioner should have hospital privileges... Whenever hospital privileges are denied, someone has caused a step to be taken which lowers the standard of practice."[4]

A brief presented in December 1960 by the Saskatchewan College of Physicians and Surgeons to the Advisory Planning Committee on Medical Care emphasized the importance of the general practitioner having access to a hospital for the care of his patients: "It is not merely illogical but medically indefensible that a general practitioner must automatically relinquish his care of his patient when the patient moves from a bed at home to one in a hospital."[5] A province-by-province survey carried out in 1958 for the College of General Practice of Canada found that in Saskatchewan general practitioners had full privileges in all hospitals except the teaching hospitals.[6]

Justice Mervyn Woods' 1963 report on hospital staff appointments corroborates the open hospital policy in Saskatchewan.[7] The report, which summarizes the testimony of 50 days of hearings into complaints of discrimination against community clinic doctors, concludes that hospital privileges were granted to duly licensed doctors in the years preceding 1962. With regard to Saint Joseph's Hospital, Estevan, Justice Woods stated, "There had never been a previous instance when the application of a candidate for staff membership was not recommended."[8]

Mr. Justice Woods heard detailed evidence concerning the manner in which applications for hospital privileges had ordinarily been processed prior to 1962 in four hospitals: Saint Joseph's Hospital in Estevan, City Hospital in Saskatoon, Regina General Hospital, and Grey Nuns' Hospital, Regina. "In each of the four hospitals, in the past," he concludes, "the record of admissions to medical staff privileges was singularly free from dispute. Privileges were readily granted to qualified physicians."[9]

In light of this, the sudden multiplicity of obstacles denying or limiting privileges for community clinic doctors could not fail to appear as discrimination.

By February 1963, many local community health associations had realized that they could not succeed in establishing or maintaining a clinic unless the hospital privileges problem could be solved. Since approaches to hospital boards had in most cases proved fruitless, it was natural that they should appeal to the provincial government through the provincial Community Health Services Association. By March, arrangements had been made for a delegation to meet with the Minister of Health and other government officials. The delegation was composed of board members of the provincial Association, doctors from the larger community clinics, and representatives from the Saskatchewan Farmers' Union and the Saskatchewan Federation of Labour.

The 22-page brief the delegation presented to the Health Minister and his officials began by reminding the Government of the sections of the Saskatoon Agreement that declared the legitimacy of community clinics. It also reminded the Government of the guarantees in the Saskatoon Agreement that community clinic doctors would be treated fairly.

The brief cited examples of communities in which health services associations had organized and taken steps toward establishing facilities for the practice of medicine by doctors who were willing to work within the medical care plan, and instances in which these efforts had been thwarted. The identities of these communities were not indicated because some of the doctors involved in the controversies continued to practise in the province[10]:

> **Community A:** The 500 family members have clinic facilities which cost them $400 a month but no doctors, hence no income. Dr.____ was with them for four days and left without notice because of pressure put upon him by other doctors.
>
> **Community B:** With 450 family memberships and facilities, a clinic was opened with one doctor. Within a few weeks the clinic was forced to close when the doctor left. The doctor left because of the pressures put upon him by the two doctors practising in ____, their

> lack of co-operation, and inability to secure hospital privileges. This has placed the local association in financial difficulties because of the commitments made for a house, furniture, equipment, etc.
>
> **Community C:** With close to 400 family memberships this clinic has opened and closed twice. The first time it closed because the doctor the local association had located was unsuitable. The second time the clinic closed because of an inability to secure hospital privileges and lack of co-operation from the medical profession there. Because facilities had been rented, these have become a financial liability during the time when the clinic is closed.
>
> **Community D:** With almost 700 members the Association has facilities for at least three doctors, with one practising at present. When Dr. _____ first went to_____ (Community D) he was put under pressure and intimidated by some of the other doctors. An offer of assistance from one doctor was withdrawn when pressure was exerted. Although Dr._____ has hospital privileges, he finds them of little value because of the refusal of other doctors to co-operate. The Association has been faced with heavy deficit financing because people are unwilling to go to Dr.____ as long as he is not in a position to look after them if they have to go to hospital.
>
> **Community E:** With 600 members, the Association has raised over $40,000 in member loans, purchased a building, and is now preparing it for a maximum of five doctors. They are planning for three doctors this year. Both of the present doctors faced delays in securing hospital privileges, and still face a refusal of co-operation by other doctors. Because of delays in securing hospital privileges the local Association has been operating with deficits throughout.

Twelve community clinics were providing services when the brief was prepared in March 1963. Of the 12, only two were not experiencing serious problems with regard to hospital privileges and/or other physicians' refusal to co-operate. Seven other local associations had made preparations for their clinics to open as soon as doctors were available. All had invested in facilities, in amounts ranging up to $40,000. All had assessed their local situation and reported that they anticipated difficulties in obtaining hospital privileges and co-operation from non-clinic doctors.

This, then, is the picture the delegation drew for the Minister of Health: a large number of Saskatchewan people, in all the cities and a sizeable proportion of the rural areas, had put forth an enormous amount of effort and invested significant amounts of money in order to establish co-operative health centres. The people had initiated and persevered in this effort in the belief that community-sponsored health centres would supplement the medical care insurance plan and make it more likely that the full benefits of the plan would be available. But the obstacles being placed in the way of the community clinics were causing virtually all community associations and their doctors serious problems in financing and in providing service, and in fact were causing the majority of the rural clinics to close down or simply not open.

The Brief went on:

> The Medical Care Insurance Act has brought about completely new conditions for the provision of medical care in Saskatchewan. It was to be expected that drastic changes in one aspect of health services would require changes in other parts of the health field, such as hospitals, if the welfare of the people is to be protected.
>
> The Saskatoon Agreement gave certain assurances, such as free choice of doctors by citizens, freedom of doctors to choose the nature of their practice, and no discrimination in the matter of hospital privileges, referrals, and co-operation between physicians.
>
> Every single one of these assurances is being violated by organized medicine in all of the areas which have, or have had, community clinics. It seems that it is entirely proper that the government, as a signatory to the Saskatoon Agreement, should concern itself with violations of these assurances.

The government responded as governments often do when they are unwilling to take decisive action.[b] It set up a commission of inquiry. On April 24, a little more than a month after the CHSA had presented its urgent plea to the government, Health Minister Allan Blakeney formally recommended to Cabinet that a commission of inquiry be set up under the Public Inquiries Act. This was the Woods Commission, already mentioned, but it was another three weeks before an Order in Council appointed Mr. Justice Mervyn Woods to head it. The Commission had the powers of a court to call witnesses and to compel them to give evidence. The assignment of the commissioner was to inquire into and report on any case referred to him by the Minister of Public Health in which complaints had been made with regard to registered physicians being refused or deprived of hospital privileges, or limited with regard to such privileges. The terms of reference included the requirement that inquiry be made as to whether the standards applied or procedures used by hospitals with regard to the applications of complainants "varied from the standards of practice which prevail or have prevailed at similar hospitals in Saskatchewan…"

The commission was welcomed by medicare supporters generally, and particularly by the citizens and doctors involved in community clinics. There were many, however, who, while appreciative that some action was being taken, were still frustrated that the action was not more direct and more likely to bring immediate results. This included community clinic patients who felt that their own health care was precarious as long as their doctor had no hospital privileges. It also included board members and doctors in those clinics which, due to financial restrictions imposed on them by the MCIC as well as obstacles placed in their way by the medical establishment, were in danger of financial collapse in a matter of months.

[b] Allan Blakeney, the Minister of Health following the doctors' strike, subsequently admitted that the Saskatoon Agreement did not help the community clinics and although it "did not lead to an abolition" of the clinics, the agreement was nonetheless "a real compromise so that the doctors were not going to organizationally oppose the establishment" of medicare, while the government agreed not "to try to change in a radical way the manner in which medical care was delivered by physicians." Though it "was never articulated," this was the underlying "compromise" of the Saskatoon Agreement. Allan Blakeney quoted in Ann Silversides, *Conversations with Champions of Medicare* (Ottawa: Canadian Federation of Nurses Unions, 2007), 29.

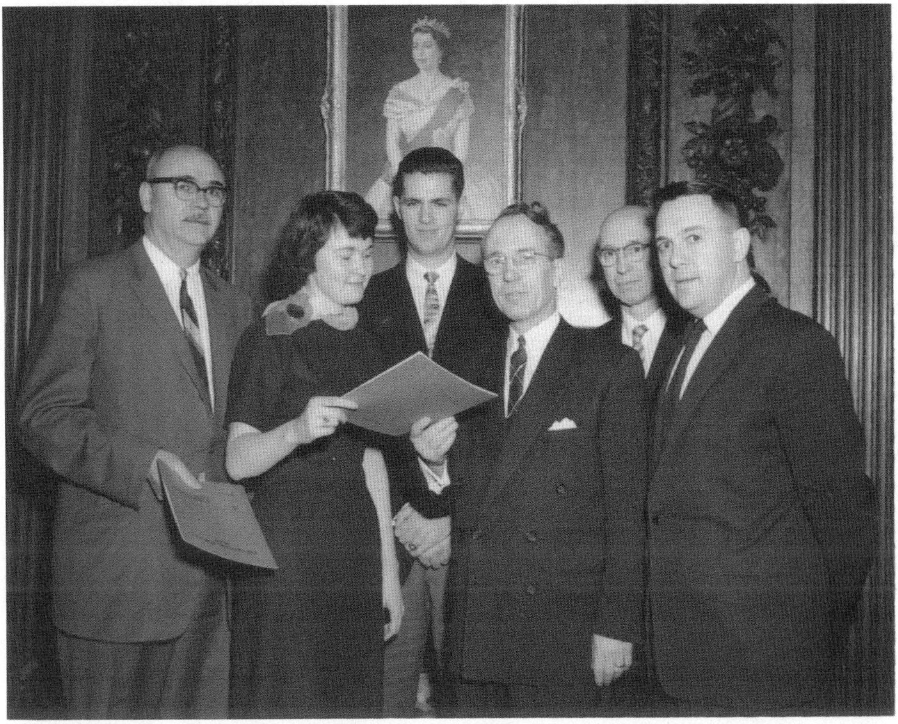

Key players in the Medicare Debate. At left, Woodrow S. Lloyd, third from right, T.C. Douglas, right, Allan Blakeney, minister of Public Health, 1962–64. All three men would be Premiers of Saskatchewan (SAB A-10,657).

In the months after the Royal Commission was set up, CHSA groups and doctors continued to encounter discrimination, both directly and indirectly.[c] Some doctors withdrew from community clinics because of the difficulty of caring for patients under the limitations imposed upon them. Some CHSA members did not patronize the doctors in the clinics they had helped to establish because of personal concerns about access to hospitals. In about 10 clinics in which doctors continued to practise despite the difficulties, and patients continued to come in despite the uncertainties, preoccupation with the hospital privileges problem prevented the development of new programs and services. Everyone agreed the problem was crucial to the progress, and possibly the survival, of the clinics. Efforts to obtain privileges for clinic doctors, and meanwhile to accommodate to the problems caused by the denial or limitation of privileges, absorbed enormous amounts of time and effort on the part of clinic boards, committees, doctors, and members. By May 1963, people were becoming increasingly frustrated.

Preoccupation with the hospital privileges situation is evident in the records of the local associations and the provincial CHSA during the early months of 1963. In February, the Regina Association set up a committee of five to work with the medical group "to get hospital privileges as quickly as possible." The boards discussed at great length

[c] John D. Bury recounts his experience with the discriminatory practices of the College in "A Physician in the Front Line of Medicare," *Canadian Bulletin of Medical History* 26, no. 2 (2009): 534–38.

actions that might be taken toward a solution. Some of the options were discussed informally with members of the Cabinet and with senior civil servants. On April 14, the Medical Directors of four community clinics met in Saskatoon to discuss the implications of the crisis and to plot a strategy. Following this meeting a series of letters from the community clinic doctors to the Premier and the Minister of Health called attention to specific evidences of discrimination.

This information lent weight to the submission made earlier to the government on behalf of all the local associations and clinics. Within 10 days of this correspondence the Cabinet had taken the first steps toward setting up the Royal Commission. At about the same time the executive of the Saskatchewan Community Health Services Association decided to wage the fight for hospital privileges publicly.

As early as the fall of 1962, the CHSA had felt it necessary to bring to the Premier's attention the various kinds of intimidation and harassment experienced by doctors who entered into negotiations with a local CHSA or with the provincial organization. At that time the latter did not attempt to document individual cases, for it was obvious that doctors who rejected offers of positions in community clinics after being visited by certain of their colleagues would not be willing to have their cases used for an exposé. Even physicians who decided to practise in community clinics in spite of threatening visitations preferred not to get involved in a public controversy with other members of the profession. Citizen groups also felt that their doctors were needed for doctoring, not for fighting legal cases.

Many specialists refused to accept referrals from community clinic doctors. Some who had agreed to accept referrals were apparently pressured later into cancelling them. In other cases, patients who were referred to doctors outside the community clinics were, when accepted, obliged to listen to a severe criticism of community clinics.

Doctors from outside Saskatchewan who had to register with the College of Physicians and Surgeons before they could practise in Saskatchewan were particularly vulnerable. Early in 1963 a doctor in England who had applied for a position in one of the community clinics wrote: "They advised me to write to the Secretary of the Saskatchewan Division of the Canadian Medical Association, which I did. In view of the information which the Secretary gave to me in his reply, I regret that I must withdraw my application for a post in the Community Health Services (Saskatchewan) Association Limited."[11]

In the early months of 1963, the College may have been a party to highly improper activities designed to deter British doctors from coming to practise in community clinics. The reports were that the names of doctors who had written to the College inquiring about placement in community clinics were given to someone in the United Kingdom who visited the doctors and attempted to discourage them. This person appeared to be acting as a representative of the Keep Our Doctors committee.

A letter introduced as evidence to the Royal Commission had been written to Dr. N. Samuels before he left England to join the Estevan community clinic by Dr. R. Inglis, president of the medical staff of Saint Joseph's Hospital in Estevan. Dr. Inglis had previously been president of the College of Physicians and Surgeons. His letter attacked the provincial government and the Medical Care Insurance Program. It criticized doctors who had come to Saskatchewan in July 1962 to serve during the withdrawal of services by most of the province's doctors. It labelled these doctors in the main as "distrustful, mercenary, and political pawns." The letter was rightly construed as an attempt by a respected member of the College of Physicians and Surgeons to discourage Dr. Samuels from coming to Saskatchewan to join a community clinic.

This impression was strengthened during the hearings by the testimony of Dr. R.W. Sutherland, Director of the Division of Hospital Administration and Standards, Department of Public Health. Dr. Inglis' letter had outlined three provisions of Saint Joseph's Hospital's by-laws which would make it difficult for Dr. Samuels to obtain hospital privileges. In fact, as Dr. Sutherland testified, none of these provisions were in the hospital by-laws.

It was a full seven months after its creation that the Woods Commission finally issued its report, and almost a year before the Government took any action to enforce equality of access for community clinic doctors.[d]

Notes

1. Regina *Leader-Post*, May 11, 1963.

2. Report of the Honourable Mr. Justice Mervyn Woods, on Hospital Staff Appointments, Regina, December 11, 1963.

3. Stan Rands, personal papers.

4. Quoted in Kenneth F. Clute, *The General Practitioner* (Toronto: University of Toronto Press, 1963), 119.

5. College of Physicians and Surgeons of Saskatchewan, "Brief to the Advisory Planning Committee on Medical Care to the Government of Saskatchewan," 80.

6. Clute, *The General Practitioner*, 121.

7. Woods Report.

8. Ibid.

9. Ibid.

10. CHSA Brief, 1963.

11. Stan Rands, personal papers.

[d] The Lloyd government took action on the recommendations of the Woods Commission just before it lost the election to the provincial Liberal Party under Ross Thatcher in March 1964.

Chapter 9
The Labour Movement and Community Clinics

The trade union movement has an impressive history of involvement in the crusade for health care for working people. In their struggle for improvement in working and living conditions, workers through their organizations have been pioneers in the fight for better health. A fascinating and important aspect of trade union history is its connection with the "social medicine" that surfaced briefly in Europe before the middle of the 19th century. Prominent among the physicians practising social medicine was Rudolf Virchow of Germany who, when asked by the government to check an epidemic, searched not for drugs or other cures but for the social conditions contributing to the spread of the disease.

In the period of political reaction that followed the crushing of the revolutions of 1848, physicians such as Virchow withdrew from the attempt to apply social remedies to socially nurtured and transmitted sickness, and concentrated instead on laboratory studies. Many of these physicians made important contributions to laboratory investigations of physical functions and bacterial infections, and Virchow himself became a founder of the science of cell pathology.

While the oppressive political regimes following 1848 sent the socially oriented physicians retreating to the laboratory, the workers of England and Western Europe had no retreat from either their hazardous jobs or their disease-ridden living conditions. Inevitably, dissension grew intense once again, and underground workers' movements, as well as overt workers' associations, were seen as threats to established authority. As one method of keeping worker dissatisfaction under control, limited reforms were implemented, including attempts at improved nutrition, sanitation, and housing.

Social historians generally give credit to trade unions and related political movements for the initiation of health insurance in Germany in the 1880s and in England and other countries in the early decades of the 20th century. But rarely is credit given to the people's movements for the improved health and lower death rates evident in the latter half of the 19th century. This oversight is due in part to the tendency among historians to interpret past events in the trade union movement from the viewpoint either of employers or of groups whose interests coincide with those of employers. But there is an additional reason in the case of the health care developments of the late 1800s.

Laboratory science began in the 1880s to show tangible results in identifying the bacteria associated with several prevalent diseases; i.e., tuberculosis, smallpox, typhus, and syphilis. This made possible some progress in the discovery of antigens effective in immunization, thus providing weapons to combat epidemics. It was natural that the decrease in rates of sickness and premature death came to be credited to these advances in scientific (i.e., laboratory) medicine, thus adding greatly to the prestige and influence of the medical profession. More careful examination, however, has revealed that most of the contemporary epidemic diseases had been checked before the development of specific vaccines, and that the major factor in the decreased rates of sickness and death was the improved conditions of life and work; i.e., cleaner water, better waste disposal, better quality housing, more and better food. The laboratory advances coinciding with the upswing in health, however, made it possible for the medical profession and its new scientific approach to take credit for developments which could more accurately be attributed to the initiatives of the working class.

These events of a hundred years ago are a help in understanding the dual role trade unions have played in regard to community clinics. On the one hand, their leadership in pushing for better and more accessible health services has been maintained. On the other hand, the mystique of the new scientific medicine and the consequent mystification of the population generally, seriously restricted the scope of trade union leadership. This limitation has taken the form of an inability to see the need for basic changes in the way medicine is practised and the way health care is delivered. The result has been a breach between organized labour's approach to workplace and environmental health on the one hand, and the treatment of individual illness on the other. Workers have been prepared to challenge their employers with regard to unsafe or unhealthy working conditions, but neither they nor the organizations representing them have dared or felt the need to challenge the care given by doctors when they or their family members are ill.

In Canada and the United States, the struggle of organized workers to win safer, healthier working conditions has been difficult and frustrating, but progress has been made. Legislation in some jurisdictions, including Saskatchewan, has recognized formally the right of working people to work under conditions that are, at the least, not obviously lethal—even the right to refuse an assignment if it involves a clear threat to a worker's life or health. These advances, along with such health-related measures as shorter hours, holidays with pay, workmen's compensation, and unemployment insurance, would not have come about without the continuing struggles of unions and labour-based political parties. Thus, the most significant steps toward preventive health have been due not to the initiatives of the medical profession or public health departments, but to the efforts of organized workers.

A second development in which trade unions have played a leading role is the increased accessibility and reduced financial demands of curative health services. By 1965, there were almost 100 union health centres in the United States and Canada, and a considerable portion of the 4,000,000 people on this continent covered by group health plans were trade unionists. Against this background it is not surprising that much of the leadership in pioneering the Saskatchewan community clinics came from trade unionists.

In the four largest urban centres, unions were well represented on the original boards of directors. It can be assumed that a proportionate number of clinic patrons and members of the urban community health associations were union members. It is also likely that they brought with them as broad a range of views about health as can be found in the general population. Among union staff members and officers, however, it seems clear that attitudes toward health problems were fairly homogeneous, and almost identical to those of the unionists who had played such a large part in the promotion of consumer-sponsored group practices during the previous decades.

Evidences of these attitudes are found in the annual briefs of the Saskatchewan Federation of Labour to the provincial government, in which the SFL strongly urged the adoption of a medical care plan, and also in the Federation's brief to the Advisory Planning Committee on Medical Care, with its strongly worded recommendations for a comprehensive medicare, group medical practice, and salaried doctors. Further evidence of these attitudes and convictions is found in the minority report submitted by the labour representative on the Advisory Planning Committee, in which he argued strongly in favour of payment by salary and against any form of utilization or deterrent fees.

The trade union movement in Saskatchewan has clearly given strong leadership in removing the financial obstacles to health care often experienced by working people, and in eliminating the pressure toward over-servicing contained in fee-for-service payments. But, like their counterparts across the continent, trade union leaders have bowed to the medical profession's dictum, "hands off medical practice."

The need for changes in the way medicine is practised has gone virtually unrecognized. One notable exception is the emphasis of some labour people on group practice. This emphasis, however, does not tackle the basic problem, since group practice only provides a framework which permits or, at best, encourages a better quality of medical care.

Recent years have seen a continuation of the tendency for trade union leaders to look sharply with one eye at financial obstacles to the accessibility of health care, but close the other eye to the need for changes in the way medicine is practised. In the latter part of the 1970s, many working people were seriously troubled by doctors opting out of the medicare plan and by the increasing use of extra billing. Trade unions in Saskatchewan, as in many parts of Canada, took a lead in organizing a broad coalition of organizations to defend medicare. In this province a number of organizations joining the coalition felt that the time was opportune to examine those aspects of the health system that people were finding unsatisfactory. Officials of the Canadian Labour Congress and of the Saskatchewan Federation of Labour actively intervened in some of the coalition meetings to ensure that activities would be limited to the questions of opting out and extra billing.

The contributions of the labour movement in the field of health care delivery have been generally characterized by the contradictory nature of labour as leaders in protest yet guardians of the status quo. The reasons for this apparent contradiction are complex. One factor is the problematic alignment of most of the trade union movement with the New Democratic Party. The negative aspects of the NDP government's policy clearly had a restraining effect on some unions. A second factor has been the growth of business unionism, which has meant an emphasis by each union on getting the best deal for its members with minimum attention to the broader social issues affecting all workers. A third factor—not specific to trade unionists—is deference to the carefully cultivated image of the doctor as a superior being whose practices and motives are beyond the competence of lay persons to evaluate.

Chapter 10
CCF-NDP Policies: Programs Implemented, Promises Made

Many criticisms of the CCF-NDP record with regard to community clinics and other areas of health care assert or imply that their weakness in performance has been a failure to carry out the declared policies of the party. On some important issues it is true that programs implemented have failed to fulfill promises made. On a more basic level, however, this comparison of performance with policy overlooks a serious aspect of the party's record. It also diverts attention from an even more serious aspect of the party's record in the field of health care. A basic feature of the party's policies and performance has been its failure to challenge the anti-social features of the capitalist health system.

A forerunner of the CCF in the province was the United Farmers of Canada, Saskatchewan Section. This organization went into provincial politics in 1930 as the Farmers' Political Association in co-operation with the Independent Labour Party. In the 13 constituencies they contested, they won 23% of the vote. These two groups, representing farmers and the less numerous urban workers, joined forces in 1931 as the Farmer-Labour Group which helped to found the national CCF in 1932. They fought the 1934 election on an explicitly socialist program which included a call for the widespread socialization of natural resources, private industry, even land. Despite the disadvanages of poverty and a hostile press, the new socialist party elected five MLAs, becoming the official opposition.

To some in the party the failure to gain power in the 1934 election was a severe disappointment. Others saw it as a successful entry into electoral politics, but recognized the need for a change of attitude. Consequently, during the remainder of the 1930s, the CCF in Saskatchewan espoused a more diluted form of socialism, often eschewing the term completely.

Despite the watering down of nationalization demands, the cause of socialized health services maintained strong support and received widespread publicity. The ideological grounds for the continued support of socialized health services must have been greatly strengthened by two distinctive developments during the 1930s and early 1940s. First, municipal doctor plans developed to the extent that, in one-third of the 303 rural municipalities as well as in 60 villages and 11 towns, doctors were working on salary and not charging their patients. In effect, a sizeable portion of the population was experiencing a local form of socialized medicine. Second, the vigorous and well-researched educational campaign of the State Hospital and Medical League developed support that appears to have gone far beyond that section of the population ordinarily supporting such parties as the CCF.

Evidence that the health plank survived the general watering down of socialist policies in the later 1930s is found in the "Handbook to the Saskatchewan CCF Platform and Policy" issued in 1937. This document declares that there is a great need for state or socialized medicine, that the health needs of the people will not be met by simply arranging for payment while the present system of practice continues, and that if we are to have prevention as well as treatment, the state must necessarily assume control. This policy statement makes it clear that the provincial party at the time saw medical insurance as inadequate, and sought an overall policy administered by a health plan with the professionals, including physicians, on salary.

The Planning Committee for Health Services of the CCF, Ontario Section, issued a similar set of objectives in 1943 but spelled them out in more detail. "Socialized Health Services—A Plan for Canada" states emphatically that Canada needs socialized medicine and not health insurance. A review of the history of state-sponsored schemes of health insurance is included in order to make the point that "such schemes are brought forward in times of social unrest with the idea of forestalling demands for widespread socialization." Similarly, in Canada, the report continues, "the two capitalist parties are offering plans for the provision of medical services at this time, when the growth of the CCF is threatening their position and privileges." The conclusion is emphatic:

> No health insurance scheme in operation or proposed to date (including the Liberal Government draft Bill on Health Insurance, which is more comprehensive that most) provides for proper redistribution and reorganization of the health services, or the integration of their activities with the other measures necessary for the attainment of community health.

The proposal proceeds to spell out details of a publicly financed and salaried health service, providing local administration jointly by law and professional persons, and health centres offering both treatment and preventive services.

There was ample ground for Saskatchewan people to assume that the party, with its socialist tradition, would bring in a health plan, not simply medical care insurance. It is not known how much circulation the Ontario proposal was given within the Saskatchewan CCF. Wide circulation was given, however, to the 1944 federal election manifesto, in which the health section was in effect a briefer version of the Ontario proposal.

It was not only within the CCF that the issue of publicly provided health care was debated well before the election campaign of 1944. As a result of urging by the CCF Opposition in the Legislature, the Liberal government of Saskatchewan in 1942 appointed a Select Special Committee on Social Security and Health Services. The public showed a keen interest in the matter, and the committee heard briefs from some 38 organizations. The representations generally fell into two categories: one group of briefs advocated state medicine with doctors on salary; the others opted for health insurance financed by contributions from the insured and with doctors paid on the basis of fee-for-service, salary, or capitation (a flat rate for each person).

After the election of 1944, some of the early actions of the new CCF government seemed to indicate that radical health policies could be expected. One of the first was the appointment of the prominent medical historian and sociologist, Dr. Henry E. Sigerist, to head a commission with the task of surveying the health needs of the province. Dr. Sigerist had studied the health programs of many countries, including the Soviet Union, and was an ardent advocate of socialized medicine. The report that his commission produced in the fall of 1944 included recommendations for health centres in rural areas, with doctors and other health professionals on salary, and with provision for a large measure of local control—an arrangement similar to the pattern intended by the community clinics of the 1960s. One outcome of the Sigerist Report was the setting up of a Health Services Planning Commission on a continuing basis. The report of this commission, brought forward in March 1945, called for a program that would be government sponsored and financed, but decentralized administratively by means of health regions. This report, too, recommended community health centres staffed by salaried doctors.

Although repeated recommendations for community health centres were ignored, a number of steps in the health field were taken by the CCF government in the years between its election in 1944 and the announcement of the Medical Care Plan in 1959. Some of these were extensions of programs which had been launched by previous governments, such as the diagnostic and treatment services for cancer which had been provided since 1930, and the mental health program started in 1931.

At the time, Saskatchewan could boast the most complete cancer registry in Canada. Only the indigent had been provided these services free of charge, but now the government extended both the programs to all citizens without charge. Improvements in the care of the mentally ill included opening further psychiatric wards in general hospitals, increasing the number of mental health clinics, developing a training program for psychiatric nurses to raise the level of care in mental institutions, and shifting the emphasis from institutional to community care.

Health regions were developed across the province, each one including a number of municipalities and staffed with full-time health personnel. An air ambulance service was established to convey rural patients to city hospitals. The two-year medical school in Saskatoon was extended to a full four-year College of Medicine, and a 500-bed University Hospital was provided. With the aid of federal grants a program of hospital construction was carried out.

Three of the new measures can be regarded as steps toward the creation of an overall health insurance system. The government undertook to pay out of general revenue the medical bills of persons who were on welfare. The Swift Current Health Region was assisted in setting up a prepaid medical and dental care program for its 50,000 residents. Most extensive of all was the hospital insurance plan of 1947, a plan later adopted by all provinces with the federal government sharing the cost after 1958.

When Premier Douglas announced in April 1959 that the Government would proceed toward a medicare plan, and when he confirmed the intention in more detail in December of the same year, he made it fairly clear that he was speaking of a medical care insurance scheme.[a] Understandably, he did not dwell on what the new scheme would not provide. There is reason to believe that many Saskatchewan people took the announcement to indicate that some form of socialized medicine would be introduced. The Premier used phrases such as, "a comprehensive medical care program that will cover all our people," and "ensure a high standard of medical care to every citizen of

[a] This sequence is recounted in A.W. Johnson, *Dream No Little Dreams: A Biography of the Douglas Government of Saskatchewan, 1944–1961* (Toronto: University of Toronto Press, 2004), 244–58.

Saskatchewan." In light of policy statements and election platforms of earlier years, these descriptions of the proposed medical plan were readily interpreted as referring to a health program administered by the provincial Government.

The major pamphlet issued by the provincial CCF to deal with the new medical care plan in the 1960 election campaign was entitled: "Your Right to Health: What will the medical care plan mean to you?" A typical paragraph ran:

> What does the Government propose? ... a comprehensive medical care program that will cover all our people and will ensure a high standard of medical care to every citizen of Saskatchewan. Why do we need a government-sponsored program? ... Only a government-sponsored program can co-ordinate a wide range of preventative and treatment services and thus make the best use of our resources. Will standards be lowered? No. In fact, a universal plan makes it possible to improve standards of care. High standards will be achieved by providing complete medical services, making good diagnostic facilities available, in both rural and urban areas, encouraging a better distribution of doctors...

In this six-page pamphlet dealing entirely with the proposed Medical Care Plan, the word "insurance" is never used in describing it. Expectations created by public descriptions of the plan have a direct bearing on the origins of the community clinic movement: the positive, almost crusading, response of many communities to the community clinic idea can be interpreted as an expression of a deep feeling on the part of many that the medicare program did not, after all the struggle, meet their expectations.

This suggestion raises a basic question. Given that the Cabinet had decided, at a lengthy meeting with its Economic Advisory Planning Board in April 1959, to embark on a medical insurance program, would it have been possible to devise a program which would meet the beyond-insurance objectives which had been referred to over so many years? In other words, can the insurance instrument be used to shape our pattern of health care delivery?

One answer can be found in the report of the Interdepartmental Committee to Study a Medical Program. This committee, set up on instructions from the Cabinet meeting of April 1959, included the most senior representatives of Public Health, Treasury, the Economic Advisory and Planning Board, and the Local Government Continuing Committee.[b] Its task was to make a thorough study of the whole area of health insurance and to report back with a detailed proposal for a universal and comprehensive Medical Care Insurance Program. At the beginning of its work this committee agreed that the Plan must go beyond insurance or it would be as limited as the sickness insurance plans of 19th-century vintage. The Committee stressed the importance of achieving three additional objectives:

(a) introducing measures to enhance the quality of services,

(b) placing emphasis on measures for prevention, and

(c) promoting the positive values of local government.

[b] These individuals included Al Johnson, Tommy Shoyama, Meyer Brownstone, William Harding, and Vince Matthews. The Interdepartmental Committee was chaired by Dr. Burns Roth, the Deputy Minister of Health. Johnson, *Dream No Little Dreams*, 244.

In accordance with these objectives, the Committee presented to the Cabinet in November 1959 a report which recommended measures to encourage group medical practice, the establishment of local health centres with doctors on salary, the involvement of local people in the administration, and extensive programs of prevention and education. Quality of care would be higher, urged the report, if doctors practised in groups and were paid by salary or capitation.

The planners for the government obviously gave a positive response to the question, "Can a new and improved form of health care delivery be brought about using the insurance mechanism?" In giving their "yes," the planners recommended features that were parallel to the objectives and nature of community clinics.

Afterword
The Unfinished Story

Maija Kagis & Susan Saunders

This book has told the unfinished story of community clinics and the work of one person in the province of Saskatchewan. We conclude by asking why a concept born in this province has had more impact elsewhere, both in Canada and throughout the world, than in its province of birth. We will also try to provide a snapshot of just what *is* the status of community clinics across the country and in this province.

While Saskatchewan was struggling to implement medicare and ordinary people were trying to establish community clinics, unionists in Sault Ste. Marie, tired of waiting for a health insurance plan, had established a clinic based on the American Health Maintenance Organization model: group insurance with a single provider.[1] It, too, was a bitter struggle, but the Group Health Centre in the Sault now serves half the population of that community; it adapted successfully to changing times and is recognized as a successful institution that provides high quality service. Fred Griffiths, the Director for some 25 years, spent two years in Saskatoon at the height of the battle over hospital privileges. He absorbed the lessons of dealing with a hostile profession, unfriendly provincial bureaucrats, and the political agendas of various Ministers of Health. The Sault, opened in 1961, survived the longest-lasting Conservative administration in the country, and became the first Health Service Organization funded on capitation when Ontario finally joined the National Medicare plan in 1968. At that time a Health Maintenance Organization, which does not provide freedom of choice of provider to its users, could not have survived, and the board and staff of the Sault negotiated a pilot Health Service Organization with the provincial government.

Today, the Sault remains a model for many health centres, for American visitors, and for trade unionists. It had a readymade community with strong ideas about what health care meant: excellent medical and ancillary service to an already defined labour community. The Sault has not yet attempted to reach out to northern Ontario, nor to Ontario's native community, but one battle at a time is probably enough.

The Saskatchewan Government was provided with a golden opportunity in 1963. If grasped, it could have avoided some of the political upheavals and general dissatisfaction expressed in 1993. With some 36 community health associations by March 1963, the government was provided with numerous communities that were supportive of drastic change in the delivery of health care. Overt government support of community health centres would not have implied immediate implementation of a "socialized" health system; rather, it could have laid the cornerstone for community-based, non-hospital health services. But in 1963 that support would have been seen as too much of a threat by a profession which had seen medicare as a death knell to all principles of freedom and democracy. The ideas nascent in this book have been adapted, adopted, and promulgated by agencies, governments, and community groups around the world. They were not just one person's ideas or ideals, but they were certainly ideas whose time had come.

In Canada, leadership for the implementation of a model system of community clinics was provided by a provincial administration. In 1967, when Castonguay and Nepveu had completed their report on health care in Quebec, they were fortunate enough to become part of the newly elected Liberal administration. Thus, not only had they been the research and policy team which recommended action to the government, they were able to take action based on their own recommendations. Unfortunately, much of the work, the planning, and the policies of Quebec have gone largely unnoticed in the rest of the country. It seems to be more appreciated in the United States, where ideas originating in Quebec are discussed in various health policy journals. Quebec is the only province in Canada, for example, in which a hospital begun by a previous administration was not built because it ran counter to the provincial plan—this in 1974 when governments still behaved as though hospitals were the solution to any and all health issues.

There have been criticisms of Quebec's plan: it was centrally implemented, there was little or no community input, and its implementation actually killed some community groups and may have encouraged a "let the government do it" attitude.[2] On the other hand, some new centres have opened without a physician, providing primary health services through nurses and social services. Physicians never controlled them: all doctors were and are on salary or contract. Some services have been bureaucratized, workers and users are not necessarily both committed to their institutions, but the process and the system are considerably more rational than that in place in any other province. Quebec has been divided into regions; the regions are responsible for the finances provided by the Ministry, but priorities and planning are done on a regional basis. And the planning is done conjointly with health and social services, since there has been recognition since the 1970s that you can't have one without the other.[3] It must be noted, however, that a far-from-left-wing administration was prepared to implement a system which could have been implemented in Saskatchewan some 10 years earlier. And without even the level of popular support that had existed for the concept in Saskatchewan in 1963.

In Nova Scotia, a Health Reform Commission recommended in 1989[4] that a network of clinics, based on a co-operative model, be set up. Meanwhile, the North End or Gottingen Street Community Health Centre provides services to a largely black, poor neighbourhood of Halifax, and, like health centres in most of Canada, struggles for its very existence. In the late 1970s the Executive Director actually negotiated a wage decrease with the physicians, and they stayed.

In Ontario, the growth of community clinics has been phenomenal, quadrupling to a total of 53 centres since 1987. Prior to the 1980s government support was perfunctory, but the efforts of tenacious community groups and the recognition that community clinics could be fiscally helpful has changed some of the provincial government's attitudes. "Ah, but they've got money," one is tempted to say. The truth is that various administrations, from Conservative through Liberal to the current NDP, have recognized that clinics provide important and necessary services to a large portion of the population, while permitting the health department to plan its own budget. Sudden cost increases caused by an over-supply of physicians and the over-doctoring of users are eliminated because the physicians are on salary. Most health centres hire doctors not only for their expertise but for their social consciences. The physicians are happy because they are well paid and enjoy normal working hours. As in Quebec, with some important difference, community clinics have become an integral part of Ontario's health policy, albeit more slowly and somewhat more painfully.

New legislation providing for payments of only 25% of the fee schedule to new physicians who choose to work in over-serviced areas and 110% to those who move to the north or other isolated areas, does not apply if the young graduates agree to work in a community health centre. They can receive full, normal salaries from the clinics, salaries which range from $70,000 to $110,000 per year.[5]

The province of Ontario has recognized, to a limited extent, that clinics provide a mechanism for predicting and controlling at least one aspect of health care costs—hospital admissions—and possibly controlling the use of new and expensive designer drugs. Thus, even if it is for mainly economic reasons, there has been slowly increasing support for community health centres. There also appears to be some recognition that community involvement in the direction its health care takes may serve to improve the health of that community as well as meeting those needs which hospitals and institutions are incapable of meeting.

In Manitoba, a network of 14 community clinics now exists, nine of various types within the city of Winnipeg and five in rural areas. One centre was born of the street clinic days of the 1970s and continues to serve a mixed population in the city of Winnipeg. Another, a women's clinic, is run by an active and overtly feminist board.[6] Provincial policy statements would appear to support the creation of more health centres, but public rhetoric and implementation are often years and dollars apart. It is worth noting, though, that Manitoba is the only province that has had the political courage to cut down on the number of spaces available in the medical school, one of the recommendations made by Barer and Stoddard in their report to the conference of Deputy Ministers of Health in June 1991.[7]

It is a sad comment on the state of health policy in Saskatchewan that the province which was once a leader in creative, courageous thinking about health services and community involvement appears to be falling behind the rest of the country. In 1994 only five community health clinics exist in the province: one in each of the three main population centres of Regina, Saskatoon, and Prince Albert, and one each in Wynyard and Lloydminister. The ability of the clinics to survive the 1980s and a hostile provincial administration forces one to respect their tenacity. One opportunity to provide a secure, long-lasting base was lost with the signing of the Saskatoon Agreement in 1962; given the political pressures of the time, it was perhaps understandable, but with 20-20 hindsight one recognizes that by caving in to the vocal and highly organized medical establishment, the NDP was attempting to serve both God and Mammon: not an easy task.

One does wonder why global or capitation funding was not made available to the community clinics until 1972. The Sault had provided an easily accessible example; the clinics were well established; most of the doctors working in them would have been happy to go on salary, since within the clinic structures they were salaried already. One wonders if within the clinics themselves there may have been an unwillingness on the part of physicians to give up that all-important control, since any global budget would have come directly to a community-based board to administer. Following the global budgeting, there was little or no allowance made for growth or health promotion programming. Some clinics, like Saskatoon, were ambitious in seeking other funding to implement programs, others relied on a policy of no growth, simply providing good quality medical and ancillary services.

In Alberta, there are only three community clinics functioning, but Alberta is also the province that has allowed the greatest inroads by American management groups. It is one of the few provinces that still collects premiums to help pay for its health services, and the Conservatives have been calling for the re-institution of user fees. The clinics all operate on a fee-for-service basis, thus facing the same problems that bedeviled Saskatchewan before global budgets were introduced. It would appear that Alberta, as it encourages more and more private medical care, is leading that part of Canadian policy which would embrace an Americanized version of health services.

In British Columbia, a brief NDP interregnum in the 1970s set up a number of health and human resource centres, most of which have disappeared, owing partly to a lack of foresight, planning, and community involvement. A few clinics continue to exist, limping along with minimal funding. As in most provinces, the political rhetoric would appear to be supportive of a community-based model, but the rhetoric is often driven by cost-control measures. It does appear that there is some willingness to attempt to implement some of the reforms suggested by the recent BC Commission on Health Care, and to involve communities in that process.

It should be noted that various aboriginal communities have now adopted a community health centre model in their own planning for health services and programs. This is taking place as programs previously run by various levels of government are devolved to local populations.

Organizing

Stan Rands's essential belief was that if you kept organizing you could build organizations that responded to the needs of people, and that you had to listen to the people who were expressing what they thought and felt. Perhaps he was guilty of a certain naïveté in not recognizing the power of the purse and the professions, often controlled by unfriendly administrations with a different political agenda.

In his review of the Kindersley experience in Chapter Seven, for example, Stan wanted people to know about both the problems and the strengths of a 'better health care system in the province. He stressed that the people in this community were extremely active in organizing their clinic. They met around kitchen tables in their own homes. They wanted to be involved in the planning of their clinic. They elected a board to oversee its operations. Stan wanted to show that people can organize to improve their conditions if given the opportunity to do so.

One can feel the pain of the Kindersley organizers when Stan describes how they felt let down by the Medical Care Insurance Commission's decision not to assist in recruiting doctors for their community. The Commission was recruiting doctors for Saskatchewan but would not find doctors for Kindersley because Kindersley was setting up a community clinic. These people, Stan tells us, had been long-time supporters of the CCF. They were proactive in supporting the Government's agenda for a compulsory, universal, publicly financed medical care plan. They were disillusioned when the government they had supported did not support them.

The Saskatoon Agreement had not only placed community boards in the position of landlords for physicians who were billing on a fee-for-service basis; it also prevented the government from assisting with the recruitment of physicians who would work in the clinics. The irony escaped no one active in the movement, least of all Stan. The government of the day consciously chose to avoid further conflict with the organized medical profession and, in so doing, promoted fee-for-service medicine and the continued dominance of the health care system by the medical establishment. Many decisions made in 1962 provide the legislative backdrop for the difficulties encountered in 1993.

It could be argued that, given an overall scarcity of MDs in Saskatchewan in the 1960s, it was important to give in to the organized profession's demands. However, the Agreement meant 10 more years of no alternatives to fee-for-service billing, it effectively stopped any development of creative health policies in the province, and it assured physician control of the health care system.

It is interesting that Kindersley did not elect an NDP candidate in the following election: NDP or Liberal, it appeared to make no difference. Of course there are other reasons for that loss, oil politics among them, but many disillusioned supporters were too tired and too dispirited to do the party work they had traditionally performed. Stan's retelling of this story is prophetic: a government that does not listen to its real supporters, who are organized at other levels, will lose that support.

Finance and Control

Saskatchewan's community clinics had to rely on fee-for-service billing in order to survive. The Saskatoon clinic did well because it had two high-billing specialists, but other clinics were not so fortunate. The boards were landlords, relying on the commitment, skills, and good will of the physicians to continue operating.

Physicians tend to seek medical solutions to social problems. Thus, the clinics opened minor surgeries, pharmacies, and optometries, but they did not hire social workers or community developers because there was no funding, and most doctors saw no reason to do so. The Medical Care Insurance Commission (MCIC) was unwilling to support adequate salaries for physicians who were prepared to work in clinics, so fee-for-service, with all its attendant difficulties, was perpetuated.

The community clinics were fighting two battles: one with the organized medical profession, the other with the very government they had been trying to support. Similar battles were going on in Ontario. The organized profession in the Sault attempted to prevent physicians from joining the new union-sponsored centre; as in Saskatchewan, they attempted to prevent newly arrived MDs from obtaining hospital privileges; they harassed both the union and the physicians working in the clinic.

The unwillingness of the provincial governments to deal quickly with the issue of salaries has meant that in recent years they have been hoist on their own petard. Canada's health care system is under attack because it is too expensive. Yet it is common knowledge that the largest expenditures are hospitals and technology, both physician-initiated, followed by physician billings. Physicians tend to bill to the level of their desired income; thus, although the number of physicians in a community may double, each physician continues to earn his or her desired salary per year. And the community which is the taxpaying base continues to see its health system eroded, made less accessible, and more intrusive in the technology it uses.

Provincial governments still spend less than 5% of the total health budget on community and public health; despite efforts to close hospitals, there has not been an even partially equivalent commitment by most provincial administrations to community based care. The rhetoric has been used, but the hard financial and legislative commitment has been lacking.

Legislation/Administration and Programs

The growth of community clinics across Canada has been hampered not only by a lack of financial support but by a lack of legislative and administrative support for their programs and infrastructure. Saskatchewan never did support anything but medical programs. Other developments were initiated through lengthy searches for "soft" money—i.e., federal or other special project grants—but clinic staff were usually so busy just keeping the wolf from the door that they were unable to apply for that soft money.

Thus, community clinics in Saskatchewan have to some extent stagnated into just another kind of group practice, providing many of the ancillary services also provided by group practices. Boards have all too often been relegated to envelope licking and fundraising. Lack of programmatic support has meant that community clinics have been unable to reach out to their communities; there is no support for infrastructure, or even the office supplies necessary for adequate community outreach. The process of working with the community one serves requires funds for meeting space, paper, and communication. Volunteers with small children do not attend meetings if they can't find a babysitter. These issues, easily dismissed individually, gain importance collectively and in an urban environment.

A movement in Saskatchewan which once attracted some 30 communities was not provided the legislative and programmatic support which would have encouraged its growth. The largest of Saskatchewan's five clinics, Saskatoon's, has developed a program to reach out to the aboriginal community in that city. Yet support for outreach programming, for community development, has not been made available within the global budgets, so much of the work must be funded through the medical budgets. The other clinics struggle to convince the provincial administration that they require legislative and programmatic support in order to meet the challenges of changing communities and economic times.

Technology

Corporations sell technology, and profit from convincing physician and consumers that technology is the answer to their health problems. The promotion of medical technology is based on the philosophy that germs cause illness. This philosophy downplays the importance of the economic, social and human causes of illness. Numerous jurisdictions are accepting the importance of environmental conditions such as adequate housing, clean water and air, fulfilling work, and other public health measures in determining population health. The health services system, and the technology inherent in it, play only a small part in people's health and longevity.

The reliance of physicians on technology is directly related to their training. Doctors are taught to remove and cure the physiological and biochemical causes of the disease. Their training, with some notable exceptions, is mostly hospital-based. They become dependent on equipment and tests for the diagnosis and treatment of illness. They are ill-equipped to deal with the human and social manifestations of illness or disease.

We have seen voluminous reports, from the American Surgeon-General in 1967 to the Black Report in Britain, which address these issues, but they seem to be ignored. Obviously, there is financial gain in promoting the germ theory, since it supports the need for new products, new technologies, and new interventions. Most recently in Canada we have seen an increase in the number of mammograms performed. Yet the head of the Canadian Breast Cancer Screening Study, Dr. Tony Miller, has questioned the value of mammography as a screening tool. Similarly, ultrasound, never proven to prevent most birth defects, has become the *sine qua non* of prenatal care. And physicians must all have coloscopes in order to diagnose and treat cervical cancer.

Many community clinics across Canada have tried to build programs around the social determinants of health, to incorporate community development and community economic development into their priorities, but these efforts often go unrecognized by professionals who have been convinced that more technology is the way to go. The community clinics have promoted the concept of primary and preventive care. It's low tech, it promotes prevention rather than intervention, and it encourages people to help themselves. Some clinics in Ontario, Quebec, and even British Columbia have used an adequate funding base to begin some real community development and try to address some of the social factors underlying human illness. One health centre in Ontario, for instance, works with immigrant Somali women in a literacy and job-training program. Volunteers in Regina have begun community information sessions on housing issues. In Montreal, a clinic provides lists of screened volunteers to visit housebound people.

Why and Where

Saskatchewan, like the rest of the country, is trying to reform and regionalize its health services. Economic pressure is forcing governments to examine the health services within their jurisdictions for accountability, efficiency, and effectiveness. Government initiatives are attempting to make geographic areas responsible not only for the provision of services, but also for limited budgets. Regionalization is being implemented in Ontario, Quebec, Newfoundland, and now Saskatchewan. Essentially, this kind of regionalization allows a central ministry to withdraw from the responsibility of providing and funding adequate services. But regionalization can, if done with community input and creative, courageous planning, provide an opportunity for communities and regions to begin to examine their health needs, their community needs. It would appear that the current (1994) administration of Saskatchewan, rather than benefitting from the experience of both its own community health centres and those in other jurisdictions, is implementing broad reforms which have only an economic justification.

It is no secret that health care reform is meant to close down many rural hospitals —often hospitals in name only, but which frequently provide some of the few employment opportunities in small communities. There has been no attempt to plan with these communities, to involve people in the discussion, to plan strategies for labour adjustment or community economic development. It has been known since the 1970s that the issue of rural hospitals would have to be confronted. The NDP has had 20 years to organize in those communities, to prevent the dislocation of the work force, to plan for alternate strategies for providing health services to the population. An obsession with a huge provincial deficit has apparently frozen the minds of planners and prevented the implementation of any programs which might ease the shock to rural communities.

Community clinics, seen as a model for health care reform since the 1972 Hastings Report, have been studiously ignored by the provincial government. In spite of 30 years' experience with a model that works, there is no strategy for using the experience and knowledge of community clinics from across Canada to improve the health and socioeconomic well-being of rural communities. Despite enormous funding problems created by fee-for-service medicine, the provincial government has been incapable of showing leadership in planning how doctors might be paid differently, or how personnel other than physicians might be used to provide health services. Fee-for-service medicine is still the norm, salaries and community clinics the exception.

We have attempted through example and discussion to analyze why community clinics have not expanded as the early founders hoped. We have pointed to two provinces where there has been some expansion, some creative policy development. We have not hidden our biases, which happen to have been Stan Rands's biases, as both of us were his students and his friends.

Stan's willingness to listen to all sides of an argument and then form his own opinion helped to sustain the clinic movement in Saskatchewan until the 1980s. Stan was adamant that communities and ordinary people had to participate in the decisions necessary to run a health centre. But democracy is painful and time consuming, and many boards have essentially remained captive to physician demands.

The tragedy is that, at one time, Saskatchewan was a Mecca for some of the brightest and the best of Canada's public service. Should the provincial government decide to support some innovative programming in health care, the brightest and the best might return to this province, either as young physicians just graduated from medical school, as nurses from urban settings seeking an adventure in the frozen west, or simply as workers willing to stake some of their savings to seek work in an exciting health care environment.

The vision espoused by the heroes of medicare and implemented by people like Stan has not, we think, died. Like prairie seeds, it lies dormant beneath the frozen ground of fiscal restraint. Stan obviously believed firmly in community organizing, and would now be rolling over in his grave were he to see what has been happening in this province over the past few years.

Or he might just smile and go on organizing, and insist that human beings—*all* human beings—are equally important and worthy of respect.

Notes

1. J. Lomas, *First and Foremost in Community Health Centres: The Centre in Sault Ste. Marie and the CHC Alternative* (Toronto: University of Toronto Press, 1985).

2. J. Godbout, "Is Consumer Control Possible in Health Care Services?" *International Journal of Health Services* 11 (1981), 151–67. F. Leseman, *Du pain et des services. La reforme de la santé et des services sociaux au Québec* (Montréal: Éditions du St-Martin, 1981). Marc Renaud, "Réforme ou illusion? Une analyse des interventions de l'État québecois dans le domaine de la santé," *Sociologie et sociétés* 9, no. 1 (1977): 127–59.

3. R. Pineault, P. La Marche, F. Champagne, A.-P. Contandriopoulos, J.-L. Denis, "The Reform of the Quebec Health Care System: Potential for Innovation," *Journal of Public Health Policy* (1993).

4. Report of the Nova Scotia Royal Commission on Health Care, *Towards a New Strategy* (Halifax, 1989).

5. Personal communication

6. Manitoba Association of Community Health Centres (MACHC), *Health Reform in Manitoba—A MACHC Perspective* (unpublished, 1993).

7. M.L. Barer and G.L. Stoddart, "Toward Integrated Medical Resource Policies for Canada," Report prepared for the federal/provincial/territorial conference of Deputy Ministers of Health (Manitoba Health, 1991).

Appendix 1
Memorandum of Agreement
Government of the Province of Saskatchewan
and
The College of Physicians and Surgeons of Saskatchewan

1. The Government of the Province of Saskatchewan has exchanged further views about the implementation of the Saskatchewan plan for universal prepaid medical care insurance with the College of Physicians and Surgeons of Saskatchewan. This exchange has resulted in agreement.

2. On the signing of this agreement, the College will ask those of its members who have withdrawn their services to resume forthwith the normal practice of medicine. In some places there may be a little delay while doctors return from a distance. This is inevitable and we ask citizens to be patient if such delays occur.

3. The Government will introduce amending legislation to the Medical Care Insurance Act, 1961, at a special session of the Legislature. The preparation of this legislation and the calling of the Legislature will take some days. The time taken to enact such legislation depends partly on the attitude of the Opposition. It is the hope of the signatories that this may be enacted as speedily as possible. The College recognizes that this responsibility rests with the Legislature as a whole and not with the Government alone. The legislation will give effect to this agreement insofar as it is necessary for it to be embodied in statute law. The amendments are set out in the appendix to this document.

4. Any universal system of medical care involving the use of public taxation must conform with normal procedures for accounting to the Legislature for the expenditure of public funds.

5. The Government believes that publicly supported medical care insurance need not and should not interfere with the rights and duties of doctors in the exercise of their profession. The doctors fear that if the government becomes their only source of income they are in danger of becoming servants of the state and not servants of their patients. We have had to find a way of combining publicly supported universal coverage with the true essentials of professional freedom. The Government and the College hope that the Medical Care Scheme outlined herein achieves this objective.

6. Citizens must be free to choose their own doctors, having regard, among other things, to the degree to which any doctor is participating in the Medical Care Scheme. Doctors also must be free to participate or not participate in the Medical Care Scheme; and they must be free to choose, within practical limits, the form their participation shall take.

7. Doctors must also be free to choose their place and nature of practice. It is not the intention of the Government to interfere with this freedom. But care must be taken in the interests of citizens and doctors alike to avoid too many doctors competing for too few patients.

8. Over the years, doctors and many of the citizens of Saskatchewan have built up voluntary, non-profit health insurance agencies. These include Group Medical Services, the Saskatoon Mutual Medical and Hospital Benefits Association and Medical Services Incorporated. It is the wish of the College that they should continue to play a part when the Medical Care Scheme comes into full operation. The College considers that they can help to protect doctors from the possible risks of having only a single source of income, and can develop additional fringe benefits under which a broader range of services can be made available to citizens on an insurance basis. Accordingly, provision has been made in the amending legislation for these agencies to participate in association with the medical care plan and for safeguarding the interests of all concerned.

9. The Government is concerned that the interests of all the citizens, when they are sick, shall be properly safeguarded, whether they belong, or do not belong to a voluntary health insurance agency. This means that the doctors shall work together as good colleagues whether they are or are not enrolled in the Medical Care Scheme. It means also that the voluntary health insurance agencies shall conduct their affairs in the highest possible standards of public business efficiency. The College is in full agreement on these points.

10. The College accordingly undertakes that the doctors will exercise no discrimination in medical treatment between citizens who belong or do not belong to voluntary health insurance schemes. But it must be remembered that, just as the individual citizen is free to choose his type of doctor, so also is the individual doctor free to elect to have only patients of one type or another.

11. There must be no discrimination against any doctor in whatsoever way he practices. In particular there must be no discrimination against any doctor in the matter of hospital privileges and attachments, referrals from one physician to another, or other professional activities involving assistance and co-operation between physicians. The College endorses this view. It is no wish of the College that there should grow up divisions between physicians and it will exercise its full influence to prevent discrimination in matters of professional practice. Accordingly, the College undertakes that in advising on applications for hospital appointments applicants shall be judged solely on their merits.

12. To safeguard the interests of patients who do not enroll with a voluntary health insurance agency, it is necessary that doctors who have chosen not to practice under the Medical Care Insurance Scheme should bill their patients in an itemized way, with a similar amount of detail as is provided at present by doctors to voluntary medical care schemes. This is in order that the Medical Care Insurance Commission may reimburse patients at 85% of the College's schedule of minimum fees.

13. To safeguard the interests of patients who choose to belong to a voluntary health insurance agency, it is necessary that the agency should be genuinely non-profit-making,

that extra billing be strictly controlled, and that it should limit its normal enrollment fees to actual administrative costs. It must furnish the Medical Care Insurance Commission with the necessary minimum data about patients treated by individual doctors, so that reimbursement may be paid by the Commission and properly accounted for. An agency must distinguish between its normal enrollment fees and premiums levied to cover the cost of fringe benefits. Finally, an agency must publish to the public full annual accounts and reports. There is no need at present to embody these details in legislation. They are matters which we trust can properly be dealt with by discussions between the agencies and the Commission. The agencies taking part in the health care scheme will have to be recognized and approved by the Government on the advice of the Commission. This is administratively necessary because the agencies will be handling public funds.

14. There may be places where few or no doctors have enrolled for direct payment by the Medical Care Insurance Commission, so that patients are denied the choice of such doctors. It is not for the Commission to appoint doctors in such places. The remedy is in the hands of the citizens themselves. They can establish premises and invite doctors who wish to enroll for direct payment to rent such premises and set up practice in them. If citizens wish advice about establishing such premises and assistance in choosing such doctors, this can be made available by the Medical Care Insurance Commission. In some small places, citizens may want a doctor where there is no medical need and where a doctor's skill would be wasted. That is why the Commission must be able to advise citizens before they make a final decision to establish premises. The interests of such enrolled doctors must be safeguarded from improper citizen pressure. The role of the citizen group in the provision of insured services must be limited to that of landlord. The only condition which the citizens can properly lay down is that the doctor or doctors in their premises shall be enrolled for direct payment. Unless abuses arise, there is no legislation needed here.

15. There may be some doctors who wish to practice without any contact whatsoever with the Medical Care Insurance Commission either directly or indirectly. The Government has no wish to interfere in any way with such practice. All that is necessary is that such doctors should make abundantly clear to their patients before care starts that they must pay their own bills and that they will not receive itemized statements.

16. To summarize the situation from the patient's point of view, he will have four choices:

> (a) He may choose a doctor who is enrolled with the Medical Care Insurance Commission for direct payment. His doctor will bill the Commission (or be otherwise paid by it) and there will be no further charge.
>
> (b) He may enroll with a voluntary health insurance agency to which he will pay an enrollment fee, and at his option a further premium to insure for additional fringe benefits. He may then choose a doctor who has entered into a service contract with the voluntary agency. This doctor will then send the bill to the agency and there will be no further charge.

(c) He may choose not to enroll with a voluntary health insurance agency, and may choose a doctor who is not enrolled with the Medical Care Insurance Commission for direct payment. His doctor will bill him at his discretion. The patient will be reimbursed up to 85% of the schedule of minimum fees by the Commission.

(d) He will be able, if he wishes, to go to a doctor who elects to practice entirely for private fees. He will then pay the full fee himself and will have no claim on the Medical Care Insurance Commission.

17. To summarize the situation from the point of view of the doctor, a doctor in Saskatchewan will be able to derive his income in four different ways:

(a) He may elect to enroll for direct payment by the Medical Care Insurance Commission. Such enrollment will be for a minimum set period of time. His payment will then be as he agrees with the Commission: by fee-for-service; by retainer and a smaller fee-for-service; or fixed remuneration only. If he practices other than by fee-for-service, he will have to keep proper records to enable the Commission to assess how much work he is doing.

(b) He may practice partly, largely, or entirely in association with one or more voluntary health insurance agencies. For patients who have enrolled with such agencies, he will submit bills at the agreed figure (at present 85% of the schedule of minimum fees). The agency will collect from the Medical Care Insurance Commission a reimbursement on a general 85% basis and pay to the doctor the amount of that reimbursement in full payment of the doctor's bill.

(c) He may practice partly, largely, or entirely outside any voluntary Medical Care Scheme, and not be enrolled for direct payment by the Medical Care Insurance Commission. He will bill such patients entirely at his own discretion. The only requirement will be the submission of his bill to his patient in an itemized form, revealing, with the patient's permission, such information as is normally given to a voluntary medical care scheme. His only possible contact with the Commission will arise if it is necessary to clear up some detail of a patient's claim to reimbursement.

(d) He may choose to practice entirely for private fees, provided that his patients also agree to make no use of the Medical Care Scheme. We expect that few doctors will choose to practice in this way, but they must be free to do so if they wish.

18. We cannot at this time assess how many doctors will decide to practice under each of these different conditions. The Government expects that enrolled doctors who elect to be paid on fixed remuneration only will be mainly in the larger centres of population and in sparsely populated areas. It expects that their total numbers will be less than the number of doctors now paid partly or wholly by salary by municipalities, but their distribution will be different. But this is speculation only. It depends on the wishes of the individual doctor himself.

19. These methods of payment are complicated, because they are designed to meet the wishes of different groups of people and different doctors. Despite this, we think they are workable. Insofar as is necessary, they will be embodied in the amending legislation. Furthermore, to reassure the doctors of the Government's good faith, the legislation will specify that the Government has no intention of establishing a full-time general salaried government medical service.

20. The Government and the College are concerned that doctors who are paid by fixed remuneration only should not be underemployed, by reason of lack of population or for any other reason. The remedy here is in the hands of the Commission. If he is under-occupied, the Commission can terminate his contract and offer him an alternative one on a fee-for-service or retainer plus a lesser fee-for-service basis.

21. It might happen in the future that too many doctors want to settle in Saskatchewan under the Medical Care Insurance Plan. This could lower medical standards by spreading work too thinly. This can always be corrected by the Commission offering only fee-for-service contracts.

22. Particular reference must be made to the medical care insurance scheme already operating in the Swift Current Health Region, and to the role of public regional boards in other health regions. The residents of the Swift Current area, the regional board, and the physicians have indicated their wish to continue with their regional plan, and the Government has already agreed to this proposal for a specified period of time, subject only to the working out of appropriate arrangements for financial assistance to the Region from the medical care fund. Such adjustments and modifications, as experience shows are necessary and as are mutually agreed upon by all concerned, will be made. With regard to the role of regional boards in other health regions, the Government feels that the time is not yet ripe to reach decisions. The College concurs in this view. Before final decisions are reached on this matter, the Government will consult with the regional boards and with the College. It must be understood, however, that in the event of a regional board, other than Swift Current, being permitted to assume the role of an approved agency, this would not prejudice the activities of existing agencies within such a region.

23. We turn now to the Medical Care Insurance Commission itself. The Commission is not intended to administer a provincial medical service. Its functions are to reimburse patients their doctor's bills, to pay directly those doctors who wish to be paid thus, and to pay bills submitted by approved voluntary agencies acting on behalf of patients and doctors. To remove the fears of the College that the Commission may assume functions other than those intended, the Government will repeal certain parts of the main Act as set out in the schedule attached to this document. The Government and the College are agreed as to the modifications needed to achieve this.

24. Both the Government and the College want to see a steady improvement in the standards of medical care throughout the province. But, in the last analysis, doctors are not made better doctors by legislation. The Government looks to the College, to the University and to the profession as a whole to maintain and raise standards of medical care. Nothing in the Saskatchewan Medical Care Scheme should hinder the developments they both desire.

25. The Government wishes the College to have full confidence in the Medical Care Insurance Commission. Accordingly, the amending legislation will add three medical members to the Commission, one a general practitioner, one a specialist, and one a representative of university medicine. The doctors to be appointed will be mutually agreed between the Government and the College. At present two members of the Commission have to be doctors. While the Government has no inherent objection to having five medical members on the Commission, they feel they must reserve the right to appoint health administrators and other citizens with wide or specialized knowledge or experience to these two places if this seems to be necessary. The Act will be adjusted appropriately. It is the wish and the hope of the Government and the College that the Commission shall function as a servant of the public and the doctors and shall not become a forum for politico-medical disputes. Goodwill between all members of the Commission must prevail if what we all desire is to be achieved.

26. There are certain other matters to be dealt with:

> (a) The Commission will have to keep certain lists for administrative purposes. The only list of doctors entitled to participate in the Saskatchewan Medical Care Insurance Scheme is the roll of the College.
>
> (b) The fees paid by the Commission will be based on the schedule of minimum fees of the College. At present these fees are fixed at 85% of the schedule. For the future any changes in the percentage or the schedule will be negotiated between the Commission and the College. Provision for negotiation, mediation and arbitration in the event of disagreement are included in the amending legislation. If mediation fails, an arbitration commission will be appointed whose findings will be binding on both sides. This commission will consist of a nominee of each party and a neutral chairman appointed by agreement or, failing agreement, by the Chief Justice of Saskatchewan.

27. The schedule of agreed amendments attached to this document has been prepared very rapidly and under great stress. There may be drafting corrections which are required to make a good Act. The College authorizes its solicitor to agree on any doubtful points in consultation with the officers of the Government to achieve the aims set out in this agreement.

28. There remains only the question of the doctors who are being or have been recruited by the Commission from Britain and elsewhere during the past weeks. The Government and the Commission must honour fully all commitments already entered into. But as soon as this agreement is signed, the Commission will cease to recruit doctors, save, of course, those needed for under-doctored areas. Where contracts have been signed but the doctors have not yet sailed, the Government will do all it can to put matters right. The Government cannot abruptly terminate the contracts of those who are already here. Some may wish to return at once and this can be arranged by mutual agreement. Some may wish to see something of Canada and Canadian medicine before they return. To them, the College extends a welcome as visitors, in and out of our hospitals. Some may wish to settle in Canada. The College will welcome them as it has

welcomed so many British doctors in the past. Inevitably there may be occasional sources of friction here and there. We would appeal to our Saskatchewan medical colleagues and our British visitors to settle their differences amicably.

29. The Medical Care Program is, we believe, a workable one. Inevitably it will have its teething troubles. The Government and the College will deal with these troubles as they arise by frank and friendly discussions together. It is in this spirit that we sign this agreement.

W.S. Lloyd, Premier, *for the* H. Dalgleish, President, *for the College of Government of Saskatchewan Physicians and Surgeons of Saskatchewan*

Witnessed:

Harry A.L.Portnuff A.M.Nicholson A.W. Johnson
W.Peacock O.Turnbull T.K.Shoyama
J.H.Brockelbank JamesL.Robertson Robert G. Ellis
W.G.Davies D.D.Tansley H.S. Lee
Allan E. Blakeney J.G. Clarkson

Saskatoon, Saskatchewan • July 23, 1962

SUPPLEMENTARY MEMORANDUM TO BE ATTACHED TO AGREEMENT EXECUTED THE 23rd DAY OF JULY 1962 AT SASKATOON, SASKATCHEWAN BETWEEN THE GOVERNMENT OF SASKATCHEWAN AND THE COLLEGE OF PHYSICIANS AND SURGEONS OF SASKATCHEWAN

There is an error in the drafting of clause 26(b) of the Agreement between the Government of Saskatchewan and the College of Physicians and Surgeons of Saskatchewan executed the 23rd day of July 1962 at Saskatoon, Saskatchewan. This error relates to provision for arbitration in clause 26(b).

It was not agreed between the parties at that time that arbitration should follow unsuccessful mediation as set out in clause 26(b) nor that resort should be had in any way to arbitration. It was also not agreed that provision should be made at that time in the amending legislation for arbitration procedure.

This error resulted from the haste, pressure and stress under which the Agreement was drafted and not from any lack of good faith by either party.

This memorandum therefore has been executed this 27th day of July 1962 at Regina, Saskatchewan by the Solicitor for the Government of Saskatchewan and the Solicitor for the College of Physicians and Surgeons of Saskatchewan to the end that it be appended to the Agreement between the parties signed the 23rd day of July 1962 at Saskatoon, Saskatchewan to make abundantly clear the actual points of agreement in clause 26(b).

J.L. Robertson, Solicitor, *College of Physicians and Surgeons of Saskatchewan* R.G. Ellis, Solicitor, *Department of Public Health, Province of Saskatchewan*

Appendix 2
Stan Rands: A Chronology

1909: Born at Fort MacLeod, Alberta. His father, a Yorkshire coal miner, had been one of the original homesteaders in the Fort MacLeod area in 1902.

1926: Graduated from MacLeod High School.

1931: Obtained a BA from the University of Alberta with First Class General Standing and Gold Medal.

1931–33: Graduate student at the University of Alberta, part-time assistant in Philosophy and Psychology Departments.

1931: Organized International Relations Club at the University of Alberta; president for two years.

1932: Awarded Tegler Research Scholarship: one year of psychological and sociological study of prisoners in Fort Saskatchewan Provincial Jail. Accepted as MA thesis and used as reference text, University of Alberta. Alberta Delegate to British-American Student Conference on International Affairs at Ann Arbor, Michigan (under Carnegie Endowment). Alberta representative on the National Executive of the Student Christian Movement.

1933: Rhodes Scholar.

1934: Obtained an Oxford diploma in Theology.

1935: Attended Summer School of the League of Nations Society at Geneva, Switzerland, including part time at Zimmer School of International Politics.

1936: Oxford BA in Philosophy, Politics, and Economics.

1937: MA (Alberta) in Psychology and Education; High School Teaching Diploma (Alberta).

1937–42: High school teaching.

1942: Member of the Northern Plains Project, a study/action group on prairie co-operatives; published *The Northern Plains in a World of Change* (Winnipeg: Gregory-Cartwright Ltd, 1942).

1942–45: Assistant Director, then Acting Director, University of Manitoba Adult Education Office.

Provincial Secretary of Citizens' Forum.

Western Regional Supervisor for the National Film Board.

1943: Married Doris Fraser of Pilot Mound, Manitoba, who was then a High School teacher at Dauphin, Manitoba.

1945: Member of the Secretariat of the Canadian delegation to the United Nations Food and Agriculture Organization, Quebec City.

1945–50: Director of Research and Reports, and Program Co-ordinator, National Film Board Distribution Department, Ottawa.

1946–48: Member of the Ottawa Civil Liberties Committee.

1947–49: Executive member of the Civil Servants Association, Ottawa.

1950–51: Provincial Executive member and health convenor, Saskatchewan Federation of Home and School Associations.

1950–51: Assistant Director, Health Education, Saskatchewan Department of Public Health.

1951–54: Assistant to the Director of Psychiatric Services, Saskatchewan.

1951–63: Assisted in a series of psychological and psychiatric institutes under the aegis of the Saskatchewan Psychological Association and the Psychiatric Services Branch, Saskatchewan Department of Public Health. These institutes included such internationally known scholars as Bruno Bettelheim and Gardner Lindzey.

1953–56: Lecturer in Psychology, University of Saskatchewan, Regina Campus.

1954–63: Deputy Director of Psychiatric Services, Saskatchewan Department of Public Health.

1957: Studied mental health programs in England, Holland and Denmark for the Saskatchewan Department of Public Health.

1958: Assistant Chairman to the Committee on Ageing, Regina.

1958–63: Member of the Psychiatric Research Committee, Saskatchewan Department of Public Health.

1959–62: Member of the Psychiatric Planning Committee, Canadian Mental Health Association.

1960–61: Member of the Health Sub-Committee of the Saskatchewan government.

1963–66: Executive Director, Community Health Services (Sask.) Association.

1965: Delegate to the national conference on the implications of the Hall Commission report.

Prepared report detailing the possibilities of greater involvement of the co-operative movement in the development of consumer sponsored clinics.

1965–66: Instructor in Psychology, University of Saskatchewan, Regina Campus.
1969–73: Acting Chairperson, Psychology Department, University of Saskatchewan, Regina Campus.

1970–71: Chairman, Regina Defence Committee (predecessor of the Regina Civil Liberties Association).

1971–74: Founding member, Regina Civil Liberties Association.

Founding member, Canada-China Friendship Association, Saskatchewan.

1971: Co-authored with Professor Les Crossman a paper on Citizen Participation in Community Clinics. The paper was commissioned by the Community Health Project, which was set up by the Health Ministers of Canada and the provinces.

1971: Associate Professor, University of Saskatchewan, Regina Campus.

1971–72: Supervised research project on "The Administration of Justice in the Courts of Original Jurisprudence in Regina," involving over 200 case studies. (Sponsored by the Regina Civil Liberties Association and funded by a Canadian Civil Liberties Association grant).

1972: Co-supervisor of a study of the Rights of Welfare Recipients in Regina. Honourary Member of the Board of the Regina Community Health Services Association.

Member of the Community Health Services Association. Member of the committee that prepared and presented to the Minister of Health (Sask.) a brief analyzing and recommending changes in the methods of financing community clinics.

1973: Presented a paper on "Some social psychological processes under Chinese Socialism" at Western Regional Conference of Committee on Socialist Studies, Calgary.

1973–74: Sabbatical: study tour of the People's Republic of China; in England did research on social movements, interviewed coal miners during a national strike, and refugees from South Africa; travelled to France, Yugoslavia, and Albania doing a comparative study of political/economic/social systems with those in China.

1976: Retired as Associate Professor, University of Regina.

1977: Professor Emeritus, University of Regina.

1976–79: Sessional Lecturer in Social Psychology at University of Regina.

1978: Co-panelist with Victor Sidel, Professor of Medicine, Albert Einstein Medical Centre, at the 15th annual convention of the Medical Committee for Human Rights, Philadelphia.

1977: Speaker at the "Oxford Debate," sponsored by the Institute for Saskatchewan Studies, facing the president of the Saskatchewan Medical Association on the topic, "Resolved that community clinics are no different than any other health service."

1979: Speaker on the health implications of the radical tradition of western Canadian politics in a conference sponsored by the Institute for Saskatchewan Studies.

1982: Public tribute at the 20th anniversary dinner of the Regina Community Clinic.

1982–85: Prepared and taught a course entitled "The Sociology of Health," for the Sociology Department at the University of Regina.

1984: Participant on the Co-operative Union of Canada's Task Force for a Health Co-operative Working Session.

1985: Member of the Board of Directors of the Community Health Services (Saskatchewan) Association Limited and a representative on the Board of Directors of the Community Health Co-operative Federation at the time of his death.

Appendix 3
Saskatchewan's Community Health Service Associations: An Historical Perspective

Gordon S. Lawson & Luc Theriault

Introduction

The province of Saskatchewan is recognized for its social security initiatives in the health services field. Saskatchewan was the first jurisdiction in North America to introduce free diagnosis and treatment for tuberculosis (1929), universal hospital insurance (1946), universal medical insurance (1962), and universal prescription drug insurance (1974–1982). Although these programs were initiatives of the provincial state, the third sector[1] was also instrumental in their establishment and continues to play an active and important role in the Saskatchewan health care system.

The first advance in the development of a universal health care system in Saskatchewan was in the field of tuberculosis treatment. In 1911 the Saskatchewan Anti-Tuberculosis League was founded in order to fight the "white plague." Beginning in 1917, this grassroots agency provided treatment and care for tuberculosis at sanatoriums it constructed and operated with provincial and federal grants and donations.

With the exception of the indigent and war veterans, all patients initially paid at least a part of the costs for their treatment; the provincial government paid a modest per-diem sum of 50¢ per patient. The cost of treatment bankrupted some patients and deterred many from seeking entry to the sanatoriums. In this context, the League mobilized popular support for free treatment. Subsequently, the Liberal government of James G. Gardiner passed legislation, effective January 1, 1929, for the provision of free diagnosis and treatment for tuberculosis, with the full costs met by a grant from the provincial government and assessments on all the province's urban and rural municipalities.[2]

The League's education campaigns and treatment programs, coupled with improved treatments, substantially reduced the province's tuberculosis rates. In 1981, in recognition of the diminishing demand for tuberculosis treatment, the League became the Saskatchewan Lung Association. In 1987 the Saskatchewan Department of Health assumed the Association's responsibility for tuberculosis treatment. The Association continues to fund research and offers an array of educational programs concerning the treatment and prevention of lung diseases.[3]

Third-sector involvement in the provision of general medical services began in 1939 with the establishment of the first of several lay-controlled medical care co-operatives in Saskatchewan. These consumer organizations provided coverage for services obtained from local doctors on a fee-for-service basis.

Saskatchewan's five Community Health Services Associations (CHSAs) are the descendants of the province's early medical service co-operatives. The CSHAs provide medical care and an array of health and social services to their members and patients at co-operative health centres that they own and operate in the cities of Regina, Saskatoon, Prince Albert and Loydminster, and in the town of Wynyard.

While the CHSAS are often cited in the literature on community health centres in Canada and are viewed by progressive health policy analysts as a model for the restructuring of the Canadian health care system, a comprehensive history of the CHSAs has yet to be written. Dennis Gruending and R.S. Reid have written commissioned histories of the Saskatoon (1973) and Regina (1988) clinics. The narrative of Stan Rands's *Privilege and Policy: A History of Community Clinics in Saskatchewan* ends in 1964 with the defeat of the New Democratic Party.

This article is an historical account of the CHSAS from their origins in Saskatchewan's nascent health care system in the early 1900s until the present. It is based on the aforementioned texts, as well as minutes, annual reports, briefs, and policy papers generously provided by the CHSAS in Regina, Saskatoon and Prince Albert.

Overview

The CHSAS are non-profit organizations incorporated under the province's Co-operatives Act or the Municipal Medical and Hospital Benefit Associations Act.[4]

The five co-operative health centres, or community clinics as they are referred to in Saskatchewan, are governed by elected boards of directors drawn exclusively from their membership of 50,000 families and individuals.[5] Membership is open to all persons over the age of 18 with the payment of a lifetime fee of $5 ($10 for families).[6]

The clinics collectively serve 75,000 patients of Saskatchewan's approximate population of 1,000,000. Once the domain of predominantly middle-class Caucasians, the clinics now also provide services to a large number of unemployed and low-income people, minorities and Aboriginal peoples. These latter groups make up the vast majority of the Lloydminster clinic's patients.[7]

The Lloydminster and Wynyard health centres provide basic primary care consisting of physician, nursing and diagnostic services. The three larger clinics in Prince Albert, Saskatoon and Regina offer a much broader range of services. In addition to the traditional paramedical services of occupational and physical therapy, pharmacy, dentistry, optometry and occupational and physical therapy, they offer nutritional information, as well as family and individual counselling. They also provide mental health services. These services are delivered through an interdisciplinary team approach to care that emphasizes prevention and health promotion. The three urban clinics also engage in a great deal of community outreach and development.[8]

The Wynyard community clinic has been active in dealing with problems and issues affecting health services in rural areas.[9]

With the exception of the Lloydminster clinic,[10] clinic physicians work on a straight salary in a group practice setting that emphasizes prevention and monitoring. This form of medical practice and remuneration contrasts sharply with the majority of the province's practicing physicians who are paid on a fee-for-service basis for medical care rendered under the Saskatchewan Medical Insurance Plan.

The CHSAs reject the biomedical model of health and illness and view social, economic, and environmental well-being as determinants of health. The Saskatoon CHSA, for example, opposed the construction of a uranium refinery at Warman, Saskatchewan (approximately 18 kilometres north of Saskatoon). More recently, the Saskatoon clinic was involved in the grass-roots campaign to defeat the Multilateral Agreement on International Investment.

In 1995 the CHSAs' combined budgets totalled $13.5 million. The majority of this funding comes from the Saskatchewan Department of Health (hereafter Saskatchewan Health). With the exception of the Lloydminster clinic, these provincial monies are provided directly to the clinics in the form of global budgets. This payment method allows the flexibility to tailor health programs to meet the needs of the CHSAs' diverse and targeted clients, such as seniors, Aboriginal peoples and those with multiple disabilities. Additional funding is provided through grants from their communities, the federal government, fees for services they render, and donations.[11]

The CHSAs are active members and contributors to the province's vibrant social economy. For instance, credit unions provide CHSAs with banking and payroll services, Co-operators Insurance provides general insurance as well as employee disability and life insurance programs, CHSAs are enrolled in the Co-operative Superannuation Plan, and retail co-operatives supply CHSAs with materials for the maintenance and operation of their facilities.[12]

The Community Health Co-operative Federation (CHCF) is the umbrella organization of the CHSAs in Saskatchewan. It is the forum through which the individual associations maintain contact and discuss mutual problems and interests. On behalf of the individual associations, the federation lobbies and negotiates with the provincial government with respect to financing, legislation and health policy; acts as a liaison body with the provincial government and other organizations (e.g. the Canadian Co-operative Association); and promotes the community clinic model on a provincial and international basis. The federation and the three urban CHSAs also provide technical and financial assistance to a women's health centre in Nicaragua.

Origins and Birth

The development of the CHSAs was the direct result of the bitter struggle to introduce a provincial medical insurance plan in Saskatchewan in 1962. Despite the opposition of organized medicine and the majority of the province's private practitioners, the Co-operative Commonwealth Federation government of T.C. Douglas and Woodrow Lloyd proceeded with its plans to implement a provincial medical insurance program. Physicians would be remunerated on a fee-for-service basis by the state for the provision of medical care to the citizens of Saskatchewan. Maintaining that such a scheme would result in political interference in the delivery of medical care and the eventual transformation of the medical profession into salaried civil servants, the leaders of the College of Physicians and Surgeons of Saskatchewan (SCPS) declared that they would not co-operate with the government plan. Furthermore, SCPS officials stated they could not guarantee the delivery of medical services after the plan's implementation date of July 1, 1962.

In this context, small groups of lay persons and several progressive physicians in Prince Albert, Saskatoon and Regina began organizing not only to provide facilities for physicians willing to provide medical services under the provincial plan, but also to develop an alternative to private fee-for-service medical practice.[13] In particular, the founders of what would become the first CHSAS wished to develop group medical practice clinics staffed by salaried doctors and other health care personnel that would strive to maintain health in addition to curing illness. The proposed clinics would be owned and administered by their lay members in cooperation with their resident physicians.

These ideas and proposals were neither new nor without precedent in Saskatchewan: they were the continuation and legacy of lay-controlled medical care programs and popular health care activism in Saskatchewan dating back to the establishment of the first municipal doctor plan in 1915. In that year, a country doctor who in the past had been unable to collect a sufficient income from his patients due to crop failures, agreed to provide medical services to the residents of the rural municipality of Sarnia for an annual salary of $2000. Through the promotional efforts of the organized farming movement, this indigenous form of lay-controlled medical care spread throughout rural Saskatchewan. By the time the CCF came to power in Saskatchewan in 1944, the residents of 101 of the province's 303 rural municipalities, 60 villages and 11 towns with a combined population of 200,000 were receiving medical services from salaried municipal doctors.[14]

In response to demands for a similar service in the cities, the provincial government enacted the Municipal Medical and Hospital Association Act in 1938. This legislation permitted any 10 or more persons to incorporate a health insurance program for its members. The first group of citizens to organize a medical service under the act, the Regina Mutual Medical Benefit Association headed by H.L. Fowler (manager of Consumers' Co-operative Refineries limited), obtained applications from eight doctors to work in a co-operative clinic that was to be staffed by salaried physicians. Foreshadowing the SCPS' reaction to those doctors who were willing to work for the CHSAs in the 1960s, the Regina District Medical Society successfully pressured all eight applicants to withdraw from the project. The co-operative organized a simple indemnity plan that provided coverage for their members' medical fees. Similar fee-for-service plans were organized in Saskatoon, Prince Albert and Melfort.[15]

Despite SCPS opposition to salary remuneration, the province's Mutual Medical and Hospital Benefit Associations, along with the Saskatchewan State Hospital and Medical League[16] and a large number of trade unions and agriculture organizations, recommended (in their briefs to the 1944 Sigerist Commission) that doctors be paid on a salary basis.[17] This was also the position of the Saskatchewan Federation of Agriculture, "representing the organized Producers and Consumers' Co-operatives.[18] But under intense pressure from the SCPS, in 1945 the new CCF government of T.C. Douglas rejected a medical services plan devised by its health planners that envisaged the expansion and development of the province's municipal doctor system into a state-salaried medical service stationed in group practice clinics with some measures for lay control.[19] The popular demand for salaried group practice clinics continued, however.

In 1946 the Saskatoon Mutual Medical and Hospital Benefit Association, with 16,000 members, announced a million-dollar plan to establish a group practice clinic staffed by salaried doctors in Saskatoon with satellite operations in neighbouring rural centres. In due course the Saskatoon District Medical Society established Medical Services Incorporated (MSI), a doctor-sponsored fee-for-service medical care plan, in order to compete with the co-operative and pre-empt its ambitious plans, which a 1951 SCPS report maintained, "threatened to completely jeopardise the future of prepaid medical care in the province and the welfare of the profession in general."[20]

By the time T.C. Douglas announced his government's plans in 1959 to establish a provincial medical services plan, MSI had experienced substantial growth and successfully deterred the expansion of both the lay medical co-operatives and the municipal doctor system. In that year, MSI had contracts with 60 rural municipalities and had a combined enrollment of 211,514 persons; and its sister organization, Regina-based Group Medical Services, had an enrolment of 69,305. In contrast, the number of municipal doctor plans had fallen from 179 contracts in 1943 to 126 in 1959. And the once thriving medical co-operatives were in decline.[21]

The growth of the doctor-sponsored plans, coupled with the decline of the municipal doctor system and medical co-operatives, emboldened the medical profession to withdraw its support for a state-financed medical care plan in 1950 and, in turn, attempt to defeat the CCF provincial medical care plan in 1962 by withholding its services. However, the Municipal Medical and Hospital Association Act was still in effect. It provided the legislative authority for groups in Prince Albert, Saskatoon, Regina and, following their example, an additional 35 communities in Saskatchewan to set up (or begin to organize) with loans from the province's credit unions, community clinics which would secure medical services during the 23-day doctor strike.

Former salaried municipal doctors, in addition to recently recruited British doctors, provided medical leadership to the clinics. Dr. Samuel Wolf, medical consultant to the provincial association of CHSAs and the first medical director of the Saskatoon CHSA, stated in a 1982 interview, "I found as a municipal doctor I could make a living on a salary instead of being paid by piecework."[22] Many of the clinic organizers maintain that it was the threat to fee-for-service medicine posed by physicians willing to work as salaried employees of community clinic boards that caused the SCPS to seek a compromise with the government and bring to an end the strike with the signing of the Saskatoon Agreement.[23] Indeed, in an address to the annual meeting of the Regina CHSA in 1987, Allan Blakeney, who had been Minister of Health during the 1962 doctors' strike, stated: "Community Clinics were in the very front line in the medicare battle of 1962. They made medicare possible."[24]

The Early Years: 1962–1964

With the end of the strike and the resumption of medical services under the government's Medical Care Insurance Act, the *raison d'être* for many of the CHSAs disappeared; accordingly, many quickly disbanded. Among others, the ideals and objectives of consumer control, group practice, preventative medicine and salaried remuneration of health care providers persisted, particularly in the larger urban centres of Regina, Prince Albert and Saskatoon. However, these groups soon discovered that the provisions of the Saskatoon Agreement did not facilitate their aspirations for an alternative to curative fee-for-service medicine; and neither would the provincial government or the Saskatchewan Medical Care Insurance Commission (SMIC), which was charged with administering the program.

First, after the CHSA doctors' unsuccessful attempts to obtain satisfactory salaries from the SMIC, in early 1963 the Commission ruled that payments to community clinic physicians had to be on a fee-for-service basis.[25]

Second, with the absence of financial aid from the provincial government, the fledging CHSAs' main revenue source was their doctors' earnings from the Medical Care Insurance Commission. At considerable personal financial sacrifice, clinic doctors gave all of their fee-for-service income to their clinic boards in return for a salary, or used part of their earnings to help establish and administer the clinics. These arrangements and financial circumstances hindered the objective of consumer participation and control.

As the CHSAs' medical personnel were providing most of the monies for the operation and expansion of the clinics, they had an equal or greater influence in their administration. In Saskatoon, this medical dominance was re-enforced by the terms of the Saskatoon Agreement which stated that "the role of the citizen group [CHSA] in the provision of insured services is to be limited to that of landlord." In this context, according to Dennis Gruending, "it was difficult for the board to accept that it had a real important role to play." The Regina CHSA's insistence on assuming administrative control led to intense and protracted disagreements and tension between the clinic's lay board and physicians. In 1967, in order to ease a debilitating debt and to eliminate its operating deficits, the Regina CHSA reluctantly handed over administrative control of its clinic to its medical staff in return for an annual rent payment and for assuming liability for accumulated back rent and loans.[26]

In addition, neither the SMIC nor the provincial government assisted the community clinics in obtaining doctors to staff their clinics.[27] In several communities well-equipped facilities stood idle for want of physicians.

The impediments to the establishment of consumer-controlled medical co-operatives posed by the Saskatoon Agreement and the provincial government's apparent unwillingness to aid the CHSAS led some of the clinic organizers to conclude that in obtaining an end to the strike and the doctors' compliance with the Medical Care Insurance Act, the government promised that it would not support the community clinic movement.

A further obstruction to the development of community clinics was the antipathy of organized medicine in Saskatchewan. Through the influence of organized medicine on hospital boards, community clinic doctors were denied hospital privileges. In response to lobbying efforts on the part of the CHSAs, the provincial government set up a Royal Commission on Hospital Staff Appointments under Justice Mervyn Woods. The Woods Commission reported in December of 1963 that clinic doctors were being unfairly discriminated against and recommended the granting of hospital privileges. Subsequently, the Hospital Standards Act was passed, providing an appeal procedure for doctors denied or delayed in obtaining hospital privileges. This legislation was repealed after the NDP lost the 1964 provincial election to the Liberals under the leadership of Ross Thatcher.[28]

1964–1971

Although the Liberal Minister of Public Health, David Steuart, ensured that clinic doctors were admitted to the province's hospitals, several policy initiatives threatened the financial solvency of the CHSAs. First, the Thatcher government introduced deterrent fees on the pretext that patients were abusing the health care system. In the view of the CHSAs, these user fees deterred proper utilization of their facilities and services. The three clinics in Regina, Saskatoon and Prince Albert mobilized the general public under the banner of "Citizens for Defense of Medicare," held protest marches, and gathered 35,000 signatures on a petition. This activism marked the beginning of the CHSAs' long history of campaigning for the preservation of medicare. To shield its members from the costs and adverse effects of the user charges, the three urban clinics set up a Mutual Protection Plan. For $7.50 (single) or $15 (family) the clinics assumed the cost of the user fees. The plan was running a surplus when these charges were discontinued by the NDP in 1970.[29]

In 1966 the government cancelled the clinics' contracts to provide minor surgery. This financial blow was followed and compounded by the discontinuation of a number of laboratory, x-ray and physiotherapy contracts. The loss of these revenue sources added to the urban clinics' burgeoning deficits and weakened the community clinic movement as a whole. In 1966 the provincial office had to close, with the association's debt of approximately $50,000 written off by Federated Co-operatives Limited and the Saskatchewan Wheat Pool. By 1972 only 10 of the 25 CHSAs that had succeeded in establishing facilities were still operating clinics. And only in the cities of Prince Albert, Saskatoon and Regina were the CHSAs successful in establishing multi-specialty group practices.[30]

The Liberals' financial assault on the CHSAs occurred despite studies by clinic physicians suggesting that the community clinics reduced government health care expenditures. Dr. Orville Hjertaas in Prince Albert, and Drs. Samuel Wolfe and Robin F. Badgley in Saskatoon found that in the community clinics the overall costs per patient were lower than those of fee-for-service practitioners; CHSA patients were less likely to be hospitalized and CHSA physicians were more productive.[31] To facilitate such studies, in 1968, the Saskatoon CHSA set up the Saskatoon Community Health Foundation, a registered charity, to provide funds for research into the delivery of medical care. While the provincial government was unmoved by such findings, these claims attracted the attention of the federal government which was then greatly concerned about the rising costs of health care in the context of its funding commitments to provincial health care plans. In the early 1970s the federal government commissioned a study to investigate the cost-effectiveness of the community clinics.[32] Since then several studies by government and non-government agencies found, by using data from Saskatchewan community clinics, that community-sponsored health centres with salaried group practice offer significant cost reductions as well as noneconomic advantages.[33]

The clinics' deficits and the restrictive funding arrangement impeded the CHSAs' original objective of utilizing the prevention and health promotion services of allied professionals along with those of physicians. As the clinics' main income source was their physicians' fee-for-service earnings, the implementation of preventive programs reduced income. Subsequently, as Dr. Hjertaas noted in 1982, preventative programs were "under-funded and under-emphasized."[34] However, the Prince Albert clinic did hire a nutritionist. And through the provision of a grant from the Milbank Foundation of New York the Saskatoon clinic was able to appoint, in the 1960s, the first social worker to be attached to a community health centre.[35] This proved to be a unique and important contribution to Canadian group practice. A study of patient referrals designed by the social worker, Genevieve Teed, and Dr. Samuel Wolf revealed that a social worker in a group practice may serve to deter or reduce some hospital stays and direct patients to other sources of aid.[36] Following the lead of the Saskatoon CHSA, the Regina and Prince Albert clinics also obtained social workers. The Saskatoon clinic was the source of further innovation and progressive health care policy with the introduction of a prescription drug plan in the late 1960s.

The Saskatoon Community Clinic and the Saskatchewan Prescription Drug Plan

Based on an analysis of the drug-prescribing habits of its physicians during the late 1960s, the Saskatoon CHSA developed a drug formulary that was used by its non-profit pharmacy. Competitive tendering, together with the increasing number of generic products from Canada's pharmaceutical industry, afforded considerable reductions in the cost of drugs prescribed by clinic doctors. These savings were brought to the NDP's attention by a board member and a clinic physician serving on the 1971 NDP election platform committee, which devised a health plank promising a publicly financed prescription drug program. After the NDP returned to power under the leadership of Allan Blakeney in 1972, the influence of the Saskatoon clinic continued, especially on the new government committee charged with devising a drug plan. The Saskatoon clinic's drug plan served as the model for the Saskatchewan Prescription Drug Program introduced in 1975—the first and, until the Progressive Conservative government reduced its coverage in the 1980s, the only universal prescription drug insurance in Canada. Because of the bulk quantities the government would centrally purchase, Saskatchewan was able to obtain drugs at very low prices for its drug insurance program.[37]

Global Budgets

The NDP's 1971 health policy also promised support for the CHSAs through the introduction of "alternative" methods of financing health services. The clinic physicians' fee-for-service billings were still regarded by the CHSAs as an unsatisfactory method of financing for reasons noted above. In August of 1971, the Regina, Saskatoon and Prince Albert clinics began what CHSA representatives in attendance have described as tough negotiations with a less than enthusiastic provincial government for a new funding arrangement. After a near breakdown in negotiations, the provincial government agreed to the introduction of global budgeting, effective March 1, 1972. Under this funding method the three urban CHSAs received a lump sum of monies based on past fee-for-service payments from the Saskatchewan Medical Insurance Commission and the Saskatchewan Hospital Insurance Plan. This arrangement allowed the community clinics to hire doctors on salaries negotiated between the clinic boards and physicians. Also included in this first budget were provisions for outpatient and social services, health education and nutrition counselling. New programs have since been added to this baseline after negotiations with the provincial government. Global budgets are negotiated on a yearly basis and are based predominantly on the utilization of clinic services over the previous year. The CHSAs retained the responsibility for raising money for land, buildings and equipment. The remaining six clinics in rural Saskatchewan continued to operate on a fee-for-service basis.

The new funding arrangements were greeted with severe condemnation by organized medicine in the province. This hostility was cited by the NDP Health minister at the time, Walter Smishek, as a reason for the provincial government's reluctance to assist the CHSAs in alleviating their crippling accumulated debt. The CHSAs felt they were instrumental in bringing to an end the 1962 doctors' strike and, therefore, were justified in receiving state assistance with the debt acquired in setting up the clinics. In a 1988 interview Smishek stated that the provincial cabinet believed the introduction of legislation to assist with the settlement of CHSA debt would have triggered a fierce protest from the SCPS. The cabinet believed the public would not have understood the need for another confrontation with the medical profession.[38]

Global budgeting brought new life to the three urban community clinics. First, in addition to facilitating salary remuneration, the relief from financial responsibility and anxiety afforded by the new funding arrangements permitted clinic doctors to concentrate on their work and quality control. The Saskatoon CHSA physicians were also able to offer medical training within the clinic in association with the medical school at the University of Saskatchewan. Medical students from across Canada chose to spend time at the Saskatoon clinic in order to learn new approaches to health care delivery.[39]

Second, the new funding arrangements allowed the clinics' consumer boards to be more involved in the decision making and administration of the clinics, as the majority of monies now came from the government directly to the CHSAs rather than from fee-for-service billings covered by the Medical Care Insurance Commission. Global budgeting also permitted the Regina CHSA to regain the administrative control of its clinic that it had ceded to the doctors in return for assuming accumulated debt. This transition occurred with some tension and growing pains. For example, Regina clinic physicians were unwilling to work for a lay board, and left with their patients. The Regina CHSA had to recruit new physicians and begin to slowly rebuild its membership and patient list.[40]

Third, with the financial stability afforded by global funding, the three urban clinics were able to expand their facilities and implement programming that, in the words of Saskatoon CHSA President Rennie Feast, they could only "dream" of in the past.[41] New programs were added and devised, based on the input of members and patients. Understanding that social problems lie at the root of many illnesses which cannot be addressed through curative measures, the Saskatoon CHSA implemented a large number of programs to deal with unplanned pregnancies, marital disputes, parenthood and childhood, unemployment, and poverty. Group therapy, chiropody, prenatal and home care programs were also established. In the area of group practice, the role of the nurse was expanded.

The Regina CHSA established counselling, nutrition and chiropody programs, as well as a senior citizen health checkup service. This new programming enabled the Regina CHSA to rebuild its membership and patient list after the exodus of doctors.42 With the introduction of a program for early detection of cancer in women, the Regina CHSA serves a large clientele of women.[43]

The Prince Albert community clinic added a social worker to its personnel and launched an extensive home care program. A wide range of health promotion programs was also introduced.[44]

Of all these new programs, the chiropody schemes had the most impact on provincial health policy. Chiropody programs were implemented in Regina and Saskatoon after a survey of their memberships revealed that foot care was sorely lacking in those communities. The Saskatoon CHSA's appeals for provincial funding support were initially rejected, although the Department of Health promised to consider funding for a pilot project. In view of the need for this service the board decided to proceed without government financing. An increase in membership assessments was implemented to finance a scheme. This program was so successful and the need so great that private practitioners in the Saskatoon area, who were traditionally opposed to the CHSAS, were sending their patients to the clinic. In this context, the Progressive Conservative government of Grant Devine, which came to power in 1982, decided to finance a province-wide chiropody program. Dr. Ritchie of the Regina Community Clinic was recruited for the position of director. Subsequently, the provincial plan, implemented in 1984, resembled the one that he had designed for the Regina CHSA.[45]

In addition to adding new programs, the three urban CHSA's also engaged in a great deal of outreach to the underprivileged in their communities, as well as in rural and northern Saskatchewan where health services have been traditionally less accessible.

In its first foray into outreach, the Regina CHSA worked with members of the North Central Community Society to establish its health centre, with clinic personnel providing services.[46] Later, the Regina Community Clinic would provide services to the rural community of Southey.

In addition to providing medical services to its satellite clinic in Canwood, which was established in 1964, the nutritionist at the Prince Albert community clinic participated in nutrition programs on five Indian reserves.[47]

The Saskatoon CHSA concentrated on providing and expanding medical service beyond its traditional middle-class membership and patients to other groups such as minorities and the poor. To this end, a satellite clinic was established in a low-income area of Saskatoon, and a community health nurse was hired. Working with local residents the Saskatoon CHSA was able to devise programs designed specifically for the needs of the area's population of new immigrants, Aboriginal people and poor people.

In 1977 the Saskatoon CHSA established an optometry program for northern Saskatchewan with a contract from the Department of Northern Saskatchewan and Health and Welfare Canada.[48]

The town of Delisle approached the Saskatoon CHSA for assistance when its hospital was closed by the provincial government in the early 1970s.[49] Subsequently, clinic personnel provided a medical, x-ray and physiotherapy service to its new Community Health and Social Services Centre. In 1980 the rural community of Waldheim approached the clinic for assistance in providing a similar service.[50] The Saskatoon CHSA also assisted the Wynyard community clinic in preparing its first global budget.

In 1980 the board of the Wynyard CHSA decided that it was time either to dissolve the association or to establish a "real" community clinic. This rural CHSA had been acting primarily as a landlord, renting office space to physicians who agreed with their ideas on medical care. In May of 1981, the Department of Health agreed to allocate funding to the clinic on a global basis on condition that it find a doctor willing to work on salary.[51]

Although the advent of global budgets allowed the CHSAs to fulfill their original objectives, they were prevented from reaching their full potential by the provincial government's fiscal conservatism. CHSA budgets grew tighter year by year and did not keep pace with inflation.[52]

1982–1991

The NDP lost the 1982 provincial election to the right-wing populist Progressive Conservative Party under the leadership of Grant Devine. Veteran board members, recalling the difficulties of the 1960s under Ross Thatcher's Liberals, feared that the CHSAs were headed for hard times.[53] In particular, they were concerned that the new government might severely alter or terminate global budgeting. This premonition proved groundless, as the anticipated assault on the clinics did not occur. The clinics' funding arrangements remained unchanged. Moreover, government funding via the Saskatchewan Hospital Services Plan (SHSP) made it possible for the Saskatoon CHSA to open a new satellite clinic (Northern Heights Clinic) in the residential suburb of River Heights.[54] However, in subsequent years, the CHSAs suffered from severe underfunding as the fiscal restraint imposed during the later years of the Blakeney administration in the health care sector continued and was more stringently applied by the Devine Conservatives.

Beginning in 1985, there was no increase in funding to health services funded by the Department of Health. In order to maintain programming and keep up with increased utilization of their services the clinics ran deficits, raised member assessments and sought more donations. However, as their representations for increased funding went unheeded and budgetary restraint continued, the CHSAs found it necessary to exercise extreme cost control measures, including staff cuts and layoffs as well as wage reductions to physicians and administrators.[55]

In this context, CHSA programming suffered. Indeed, the Regina clinic had to discontinue some programs completely and was unable to introduce new ones. Nor could it serve all the people who wanted access to its facilities and services.[56]

The Saskatoon CHSA initially placed its programming plans on hold, but later resolved to proceed with some new programs because they were urgently needed in the community and would improve the profile of the clinic and encourage its use. In addition to more counselling programs, a health maintenance program for women aged 45–64 was introduced. Moreover, after the province's universal drug plan was discontinued, the Saskatoon CHSA offered financial assistance to those who could not afford prescription drugs. To support these initiatives and to continue to improve and experiment with better methods of health services delivery the Saskatoon CHSA increasingly relied on its Community Health Foundation, which in 1984–85 received approval from Revenue Canada to receive donations for projects other than research.[57]

The Prince Albert clinic also found it difficult to add new or expanded programs, but managed to do so by relying on voluntary funding.[58]

The CHSAs were wary of publicly criticizing the government's health policy, owing to their dependence on government funding and the fact that their funding arrangements with SHSP had 30-day cancellation clauses. However, as budgetary restraints continued and included the discontinuation of the Saskatchewan Prescription Drug Plan that the Saskatoon community clinic had pioneered, as well as the children's dental plan introduced by the NDP in 1974, the CHSAs decided that the health funding cuts had to be met with strong protests. In cooperation with the Saskatchewan Health Coalition and CUPE, the Community Health Co-operative Federation (CHCF) held a well-attended and publicized protest march in Regina on June 20, 1987; a similar march had taken place in Saskatoon on June 17, 1987.[59]

Adding to the clinics' frustrations with the Devine government was the suppression of a 1983 Saskatchewan Health survey of the Saskatoon and Prince Albert CHSAs revealing that their services led to lower per capita health care costs, lower prescription drug utilization, fewer hospitalizations and shorter hospital stays. It was only after intense lobbying by the CHSAs that the government released the results of this study in 1989. As with the earlier studies, the CHSAs hoped that these findings would result in increased funding and recognition. While there were several minor changes to funding policy in 1991 that afforded greater flexibility and improved the clinics' financial position, there were no increases in funding. Moreover, the Commission on Directions in Health Care, appointed by the provincial government in 1989 to review Saskatchewan's health care system and make recommendations for its reform, virtually ignored the community clinics. The Commission's final report simply stated that the legal and funding status of the community clinics should be reviewed and clarified by another committee.

Wellness and the NDP: 1992–1998

In mid January 1992, after the NDP had been returned to power, CHCF representatives met with the minister of Health, Louise Simard, for the first time in 10 years. They were assured of the new government's commitment to community based alternatives in care and delivery, and of a continuing role for community clinics in health reform.[60] This positive reception, coupled with the unveiling of the provincial government's health reform agenda in February, made the CHSAs optimistic that the financial and legislative security they had sought for so long would now finally be realized.

The new government's health reform agenda entailed the closure and conversion of approximately 51 rural hospitals into community health centres, and the establishment of elected district health boards responsible for the planning, administration and delivery of services in their jurisdictions based on community needs assessments. These structural reforms were to be accompanied by a new holistic approach to health and illness, the so-called "wellness" model, emphasizing disease prevention, health promotion, consumer participation, the integration of institutional, community-based and preventive services, and the reduction of health inequities among low-income and Aboriginal peoples.[61]

As the CHSAs observed, the government health reform program and the wellness model were consistent with the community clinics' founding principles that they had sought to embody and promote from their inception. Accordingly, despite reservations about their place in this new order and their future relationship with the proposed district health boards, the CHSAs enthusiastically endorsed the government's reform initiatives and declared that they would cooperate with the provincial government and the new district health boards in reforming the province's health care system. The Prince Albert CHSA even considered promoting the government's health care reforms to a skeptical public. In its 1992 annual report the board of directors noted that the co-operative health centre "has a role to play to help allay the fears and misinformation [re: wellness], which are founded on lack of understanding."[62]

In Prince Albert, the CHSA assumed a leadership role in the development of the local health board. Clinic staff, including Stan Rice (administrator of the Prince Albert CHSA and a long-time leader of the community clinic movement) and Paige Finney

(Program Development Officer), were seconded to the new health board to formulate policy and get programming off the ground. In 1993 Stan Rice accepted a permanent position as Chief Executive Administrator of the Prince Albert Health Board. The CHSA representatives also contributed to various working groups and committees set up to examine and devise existing and new community-based services for Prince Albert.[63] In addition, the Prince Albert Community Clinic shared information and provided assistance with purchasing, laundry services, and realizing efficiencies. Through such cooperation with the local health board, the clinic's medical director foresaw an "enhancement of our services."[64]

Throughout its active cooperation and participation in the formation of the Prince Albert Health District, the clinic's administrators and physicians remained committed to maintaining their autonomy. Accordingly, it shared with the other CHSAs a profound disappointment and concern when informed in 1994 that the provincial government intended to transfer funding responsibility for the community clinics over to the district health boards.[65]

In a discussion paper concerning the proposed funding transfer, the Saskatoon CHSA observed that the district health boards had "shown little interest in, or support for our services and community based services in general ... they appear to be primarily focused on the acute care agenda."[66] Indeed, when representatives of the Regina CHSA met with the Regina District Health Board for the first time in November 1992 they found that district health board members had "very little knowledge of the community clinic model."[67] In this context, the CHSAs feared for their autonomy and ability to provide the quality and variety of services made possible by global budgets from Saskatchewan Health. In addition, the Saskatoon CHSA, the most "politically active" of the community clinics, feared that funding control might compromise its capacity to independently advocate for the health care interests of its members and patients. The Saskatoon clinic would risk conflict with the district health board due to advocacy positions taken on behalf of clinic members, which in turn might affect the district health board's willingness to support clinic programs.[68] Therefore, the CHSAs were determined to resist the proposed funding transfer.

In November of 1994 the CHCF presented a brief to the provincial government requesting that Saskatchewan Health continue to fund CHSAs directly, and that any decision to transfer funding responsibility to district health boards be deferred for a minimum of three years. Should the provincial government proceed to transfer fiscal responsibility for CHSAs, legislation and/or regulations protecting their health care delivery models and funding should be established prior to the transfer. The Federation reiterated its support for health care reform and its commitment to working with the district health boards to provide effective, economic, and efficient health care delivery. This could be accomplished through affiliation agreements addressing the involvement of CHSAs in joint needs assessment, planning, coordination and service delivery.[69] The minister promised to review the proposed transfer and committed global funding under Saskatchewan Health for another year.

In subsequent years, while Saskatchewan Health continued to provide global budgets on a year-by-year basis, it appeared that the clinics would eventually fall under the jurisdiction of district health boards.[70] However, their campaign of resistance seems to have succeeded.

In 1997, federation representatives adopted a set of principles which, they hoped, would form the basis of a tripartite agreement with Saskatchewan Health and the district health boards. These principles are: 1) the CHSAs will retain their autonomy and governance models; 2) Saskatchewan Health will continue to provide global funding for the delivery of primary health care for the populations served by the clinics; 3) co-operative health centres will seek incremental funding from district health boards for additional community needs, and they will consult with the boards before introducing new community programming; and 4) the district health boards and co-operative health centres will work together to identify and address health needs in the communities they serve.[71]

When the Federation met with Saskatchewan Health in April 1998, it was agreed to set up a committee of representatives from the three parties to fast-track the signing of this agreement by the end of June 1998. This agreement has yet to be ratified.[72]

In the meantime, the CHSAs have sought to strengthen their relationships with the district health boards. These relationships vary a great deal and have evolved differently from district to district.

In terms of funding, the current NDP administration has restored some of the revenue the CHSAs were deprived of during the Devine administration. There have been no new cuts, and Saskatchewan Health has provided some modest increases to the CHSA global budgets. However, these funding increases were considerably less than inflationary costs and much lower than those granted to the district health boards. They could by no means meet the increasing demands for services, let alone alleviate the clinics' lingering financing difficulties.[73]

It is only through further cost control and ingenuity that the community clinics have been able to maintain their impressive array of health and social services. At the same time, and despite limited resources, the CHSAs continue to respond to calls for assistance from communities that lost services as the province closed health care facilities. The CHSAs continue to reach out to alleviate the health care needs of the underprivileged in these communities, as the following examples indicate.

After the rural community of Birch Hills lost its hospital and, in turn, its resident physician as part of the closure of 51 rural hospitals throughout the province, the Prince Albert CHSA was approached and agreed to provide medical and other health services for its new health centre. The Prince Albert CHSA continues to provide physician and health services to the rural communities of Canwood and Birch Hills, while the communities of Delisle and Borden are served by the Saskatoon CHSA. The Saskatoon CHSA doubled the space at its westside clinic in order to expand and enrich programming for its patients, many of whom suffered from discrimination, unemployment and poverty. In Regina, the CHSA chose a tradition-ally underserved area of the city for the relocation of its main clinic in 1996.[74]

Adding to the CHSAs' disappointment and unfulfilled expectations has been the provincial government's health centre policy. The Federation had hoped that health centres would be developed along the lines of Saskatchewan's community clinics with a strong emphasis on community ownership and consumer involvement in their design and delivery. However, there was little commitment or interest amongst district health boards, Saskatchewan Health, or the Saskatchewan Economic and Co-operative Development Branch in the grass-roots development of co-operative health centres.

Undeterred from its vision of expanding its model of health care delivery in Saskatchewan, the Federation has turned to the larger co-operative movement in the province to facilitate this objective. The CHSAs have requested that the co-operative sector assist in identifying, financing and working with communities interested in developing co-operative health centres. As a first step towards this initiative, the co-operative sector has been asked to fund the appointment and activities of a co-operative health centre developer for a three-year project.[75]

Conclusion

Saskatchewan's CHSAs are the legacy and expression of the popular demand for consumer control of health services and salaried group practice clinics in the province dating back to the early 1900s. Like the Saskatchewan Anti-Tuberculosis League, these third-sector agencies have been the prime movers and source of health reform in Saskatchewan. They were instrumental in the establishment of state-financed medical and prescription drug insurance in Saskatchewan. Since then they have led the struggle to defend and prevent the erosion of these social security programs. Despite the lack of political commitment and legislative legitimacy, inadequate funding, the difficulty in attracting medical personnel and the opposition of organized medicine, the CHSAs have been able to offer an alternative to traditional curative medicine. Through salaried group practice and consumer participation, the CHSAs provide quality and innovative health and social services to the citizens of Saskatchewan. The CHSAs have each faced similar adversities and have come together to achieve a mutual objective; yet, owing to the diversity of patients, member-ships and communities, each CHSA is distinct and has its own unique historical place in the development of health care in Saskatchewan.

Notes

We are grateful to Human Resources Development Canada for supporting the Saskatchewan Social Economy Research Project and helping to make this article possible. We wish also to thank the Social Policy Research Unit, Faculty of Social Work, University of Regina, for its contributions to various phases of research and its production assistance. Originally published in Prairie Forum 24, no. 2 (1999): 251–68.

1. Many organizations in society are neither private-sector businesses run for a profit nor government-owned state corporations or agencies. They are rather independent organizations created to provide a service either to the public or to a defined membership. We follow here the Canadian tradition in referring to such organizations as belonging to the "third sector" of the economy. In the United Kingdom the term "voluntary sector" tends to be used for these organizations, while in France and in Quebec the term *économie sociale* ("social economy") is more common.

2. C. Stuart Houston, *R. G. Ferguson: CrusaderAgainst Tuberculosis* (Toronto and Oxford: Hannah Institute & Dundurn Press, 1991), 72, 81–82.

3. Ibid., 185.

4. Community Health Co-operative Federation Limited, "Proposal for the Involvement of the Saskatchewan Co-operative Community in the Development of Co-operative Health Centres in Saskatchewan, October 20, 1997," 3.

5. Ibid.

6. The Loydminster clinic is currently exploring the possibility of granting membership to anyone who uses the clinic's services. Telephone interview with Dal Windram, administrator of the Lloydminster CHSA.

7. Ibid.

8. Community Health Co-operative Federation Limited," 3.

9. The Community Health Co-operative Federation of Saskatchewan, "Brief to the Saskatchewan Commission on Directions in Health Care, March 1989," 57.

10. The physicians providing medical care at the Lloydminster clinic bill the Saskatchewan and Alberta governments for services rendered on a fee-for-service basis. The current administrator of the Lloydminster community clinic is optimistic that several physicians who rent office space from CHSA will accept a salary arrangement. The city of Lloydminster straddles the Alberta and Saskatchewan provincial borders. The Lloydminster clinic provides services to patients and members in both jurisdictions.

11. Denise Albrecht and Patrick Lapointe, "Community Health Centres in Canada: In a Land of Opportunities and Threats," presented to International Conference on Community Health Centres, December 3–6, 1995.

12. Community Health Co-operative Federation Limited, "Proposal," 3.

13. Dennis Gruending, *The First 10 Years* (Saskatoon: Community Health Services Association, 1973), 7; Prince Albert Community Clinic (hereafter PACC), Minutes, May 26, 1962; Margaret Hughes, *A Biography: The Community Health Center Regina* (Regina: Community Health Services Association (Regina) Ltd., 1977), 4.

14. Seymour Martin Lipsett, *Agrarian Socialism: The Co-operative Commonwealth in Saskatchewan* (Berkley: University of California Press, 1950), 228.

15. Stan Rands, *Privilege and Policy: A History of Community Clinics in Saskatchewan* (Saskatoon: Community Health Co-operative Federation, 1994), 25; Robin F. Badgley and Samuel Wolfe, *Doctors' Strike: Medical Care and Conflict in Saskatchewan* (Toronto: Macmillan, 1967), 16–17.

16. The SHML was a confederation of voluntary and governmental organizations including homemakers clubs, fraternal societies, church and farm organizations, the Saskatchewan Teachers Federation, co-operative groups, 120 rural municipalities, 6 cities, 24 towns and 56 villages. Established in the city of Prince Albert in 1936, the League lobbied the provincial government to establish a comprehensive medical hospital services plan. It was a staunch opponent of fee for-service remuneration.

17. Gordon Stewart Lawson, "The Co-operative Commonwealth Federation, Health Care Reform and Physician Remuneration in the Province of Saskatchewan, 1915–1949" (Master's thesis, University of Regina, 1998), 58–61.

18. Ibid., 59.

19. Ibid.,102–11.

20. C.D. Naylor, *Private Practice, Public Payment: Canadian Medicine and the Politics of Health Insurance, 1911–1966* (Kingston and Montreal: McGill-Queen's University Press, 1986), 149; Malcolm G. Taylor, *Health Insurance and Canadian Public Policy: The Seven Decisions that Created the Canadian Health Insurance System* (Montreal: McGill-Queen's University Press, 1978), 260.

21. Taylor, *Health Insurance and Canadian Public Policy*, 260.

22. "Saskatoon Doctor Recalls Early Days of Medicare," *Saskatoon StarPhoenix*, June 7, 1982.

23. Benjamin G. Smillie, "Foreword" to Rands, *Privilege and Policy*, 10–14.

24. Reid, *More than Medicare* (Regina: Community Health Services Association (Regina) Ltd., 1988), 44.

25. Rands, *Privilege and Policy*, 75.

26. Prince Albert Community Clinic (hereafter FACC) , O.K. Hjertaas, Medical Director's

Report, April 24, 1972, p. 9; Gruending, *The First 10 Years*, 21; Reid, *More than Medicare*, 18–21, 31–32; Hughes, *The Community Health Center Regina*, 20.

27. Rands, *Privilege and Policy*, 66–70.

28. Ibid., 83–93; Gruending, *The First 10 Years*, 17.

29. Ibid., 20.

30. Reid, *More than Medicare*, 29; D.O. Anderson, "The Feasibility of a Study of the Community Clinics and Other Group Practices in Saskatchewan." Report Commissioned by the Director of Medical Care, Department of National Health and Welfare, November 1, 1969, pp. 15–16; Gruending, The First Ten Years, 10, 19.

31. PACC, O.K. Hjertaas, Medical Director's Report, April 24, 1972; O.K. Hjertaas, "A Study of Health Care Economics in a Consumer Sponsored Group Practice in Saskatchewan," *Group Health and Welfare News*, February 10, 1969; S. Wolfe et al., "A Description and Analysis of the Work of a Group of Doctors," *Milbank Memorial Fund Quarterly* 46 (1968): 103.

32. See D.O. Anderson and A. Crichton, *What Price Group Practice?* (Vancouver: Mitchell Press, 1973).

33. See for example, Douglas E. Angus and Pran Manga, *Co-op/Consumer Sponsored Health Care Delivery Effectiveness* (Ottawa: Canadian Co-operative Association, 1990).

34. PACC, O.K. Hjertaas, "Retirement Report to Board," April 14, 1982, p. 9.

35. Community Health Services Association, Saskatoon (hereafter CHSAS), Account of the 20th anniversary celebration of Medicare and Community Health Services (Saskatoon) Association, June 5, 1982.

36. Ibid., 27; Samuel Wolfe and Genevieve Teed, " A Study of the Work of a Medical Social Worker in a Group Medical Practice," *Canadian Medical Association Journal*, May 27, 1967.

37. CHSAS, Brenda Mager, Judy Brady and John Bury, "In Memoriam—The Saskatchewan Prescription Drug Plan," Focus 23, no. 4 (July–August 1987); Jim Harding, "The Welfare State as a Therapeutic State: The Saskatchewan Prescription Drug Plan 1974–1982," in Jim Harding, *Social Policy and Social Justice: The NDP Government in Saskatchewan during the Blakeney Years* (Waterloo: Wilfrid Laurier University Press, 1994), 92.

38. Reid, *More than Medicare*, 44.

39. CHSAS, Margaret Mahood, Medical Director, "[Report] for the Eleventh Annual Meeting, March 30, 1974."

40. T. Kue Young, "Lay-Professional Conflict in a Canadian Community Health Centre: A Case Report," in Coburn, D'Arcy, New and Torrance (eds.), *Health and Canadian Society: Sociological Perspectives* (Toronto: Fitzhenry & Whiteside Limited, 1981), 307–9.

41. CHSAS, Rennie Fast, "Board Report," *Focus*, January–February 1994.

42. Reid, *More than Medicare*, 45.

43. The Community Health Co-operative Federation of Saskatchewan, Brief to the Saskatchewan Commission on Directions in Health Care, March 1989, p. 56.

44. PACC, O.K. Hjertaas, "Retirement Report to Board," April 14, 1982, p. 8.

45. CHSAS, Minutes of Membership Meeting Held at Western Coop College, November 15, 1974; CHSAS, Clinical Co-ordinators Annual Report 1980; Reid, More than Medicare, 54.

46. Ibid., 53.

47. PACC, Linda Jensen, Presentation to Honourable Justice Emmett M. Hall, At the Co-operative Health Centre Prince Albert, Saskatchewan, January 29, 1980, on nutrition education programs, p. 3.

48. CHSAS, "Clinical Coordinator's Report-1977–1978," *Focus* 14, no. 3 (May–June 1978).

49. CHSAS, "Summary of Annual Meeting, CHSA, held Wednesday, January 28, 1981 at the Lawson Heights School."

50. CHSAS, John McConnel, "Director's Report," *Focus* 16, no. 3 (May–June 1980).

51. Wendy Roy, "Staying Healthy Co-operatively," *Western People*, June 22, 1982.

52. Reid, *More than Medicare*, 54.

53. CHSA, President's Message to the Annual Meeting of Community Health Services (Saskatoon) Association Limited, June 4, 1983.

54. Ibid.

55. CHSAS, C.A. Robson, President's Report to the 25th Annual Meeting of C.H.S. (Saskatoon) Ass'n Ltd., June 3, 1987; Community Health Services Association, Regina (hereafter CHSAR), Tom Marwick, "Executive Director's Report," *Pulse* 19 (June 1988); Reid, *More than Medicare*, 55; CHSAS, Trevor Shepstone, Report to Annual Meeting, June 12, 1987; CHSAS, *Focus* 21, no. 2 (March–April 1985); CHSAS, Judith Martin, Administrator's Report, Annual General Meeting, June 15, 1988.

56. CHSAR, *Pulse* 19 (June 1988); *Pulse* 20 (June 1989); Reid, *More than Medicare*, 45.

57. CHSAS, Report on 1987 AGM: Resolutions and Follow-Up in the Order as Voted on the 1987 AGM; CHSAS, Trevor Shepstone, Report to Annual Meeting, June 12, 1985; CHSAS, Administrator's Report Annual General Meeting, June 15, 1988; CA. Robson, President's Report to the 25th Annual Meeting of C.H.S. (Saskatoon) Ass'n Ltd., June 3, 1987; CHSAS, *Focus* 21, no. 6 (November–December 1985).

58. PACC, Stan Rice, "Administrator's Annual Report," June 8, 1988.

59. CHSAS, C.A. Robinson, President's Report Annual General Meeting, June 15, 1988.

60. CHSAR, *Pulse* 23 (June 1992).

61. Province of Saskatchewan, *A Saskatchewan Vision for Health: A Framework for Change* (Regina: Saskatchewan Health, 1992).

62. PACC, Board of Director's Report, 1992.

63. PACC, Lydia Uhlik, Administrator's Report, 1993.

64. PACC, Medical Directors Report, circa 1992.

65. CHSAS, Discussion Paper: Community Health Services Associations Affiliation District Health Boards (Provided By Community Health Services (Saskatoon) Members), October 7, 1994; CHSAS, Annual Report (1993–94).

66. CHSAS, Discussion Paper: Community Health Services Associations Affiliation District Health Boards (Provided By Community Health Services (Saskatoon) Members), October 7, 1994.

67. Ibid.; CHSA, Annual Report, 1993.

68. CHSAS, Discussion Paper, supra, October 7, 1995.

69. CHCF, Brief to the Cabinet of the Government of Saskatchewan, November 1994.

70. CHSAR, Annual Report, 1996.

71. CHSAR, Annual Report, 1998.

72. Ibid.

73. CHSAS, Annual Report, 1993–1994; CHSAR, Annual Report, 1993.

74. CHSAS, Annual Report, 1993–1994; PACC, Prince Albert Community Clinic Medical Group Annual Report: for the 1998 Annual General Meeting; PACC, Dr. R.J. Unsworth,

Medical Director's Report, 1993; Interview with Donna Braun, Community Relations, CHSAR, July 1998.

75. Community Health Co-operative Federation Limited, Proposal for the Involvement of the Saskatchewan Co-operative Community in the Development of Co-operative Health Centres in Saskatchewan, October 20, 1997, p. 5.

Afterword to the 2012 Edition: Co-operatives and Consumer Control of Health Care Services: A Look 50 Years Later

Catherine Leviten-Reid

In his writing and his work, Stan Rands argued for a universal health care system that featured consumer control over the services being delivered. In Saskatchewan, this control materialized through the formation of co-operatives, an organizational form that, as Rands explained in chapter one, already had a long tradition in the province when the community clinics emerged in 1962.

What is the status of consumer-controlled health co-operatives 50 years after the first community clinics were organized in Saskatchewan? And what does their future hold? To address these questions, this chapter will provide descriptive information on the number and nature of health co-operatives across the country and discuss overall trends with regard to consumer involvement within this organizational form. This chapter will also address the challenges and opportunities that lay ahead for these associations. First, however, some background information will be provided on the nature of co-operative organizations and consumer control.

The Co-operative Form and Consumer Control

Since the vision of Stan Rands was to transform the provision of health care services from a private service exchanged in the marketplace to a universal service provided as a public good, the term "consumer" control over the services provided by these co-operatives seems perhaps a misnomer. Indeed, these organizations remain fiercely committed to universal and publicly funded health care delivery.[1] Moreover, unlike their market-oriented counterparts, such as credit unions and co-operative food stores, community clinics in Saskatchewan are non-profit co-operatives and they receive mostly government funding to cover the cost of their operations. Yet "consumer" control is used for two reasons: the term is used in the health care and co-operative literatures in the context of the consumer sponsorship of health care services,[2] and because early clinic organizers used the term, including Rands in this volume.[3]

Co-operatives allow for consumer control of the goods or services they provide through the principle of "democratic member control"—a characteristic that is recognized internationally as being a core feature of this organizational type.[4] This principle means that members have the opportunity to participate equally and actively in the affairs of their co-operatives. Democratic member control is not only a characteristic of all co-operatives; it is enshrined in federal[5] and provincial[6] legislation pertaining to the co-operative form as well as the by-laws of these organizations.[7]

The memberships of the four active community clinics in Saskatchewan consist of those who use the services of the associations. Consumer control is achieved in the Prince Albert, Regina, Saskatoon and Wynyard clinics because these members have the opportunity to vote—on a one-person, one-vote basis—for who will be on the board and may choose to run for the board themselves.[8] Board functions include approving the yearly budget, overseeing and evaluating the work of the executive director, and strategic planning to set priorities for the health organizations. Financial statements are presented to members at annual meetings and approved by them, as are reports on the activities of the clinics which are delivered by staff, management and directors.[9] Members' meetings are also venues where users of the co-operatives' services may bring forward resolutions for discussion and debate; current examples from the Saskatoon Community Clinic include resolving that the organization should actively encourage the federal government to invest in anti-smoking initiatives, and that the organization should advocate for more public funding for social housing, with the understanding that housing is a social determinant of health.[10]

To be sure, the literature on co-operatives and social economy organizations more broadly is replete with discussion and debate regarding how much input and direction boards of directors, in practice, are able to provide the organizations that they govern; the debate typically focuses on the role that senior staff members play in organizational decision-making versus the board of directors.[11] Further, scholars and practitioners often bemoan low turnout rates at the members' meetings of co-operatives of all kinds.[12] And while in practice there is indeed variation among all co-operatives (and across time within single co-operatives) regarding active participation in governance, consumer control is still embedded in the co-operative form. If a members' meeting is poorly attended, the structure of the meeting is in place so that when users feel they need to voice concerns to current directors, elect different board members, or run for the board themselves, a mechanism is in place for them to do so. Similarly, members of a co-operative have the opportunity to replace an inactive board of directors with one that is more involved in the affairs of the organization.

Health Co-operatives in Canada: A Current Picture

An annual survey conducted by the Rural and Co-operatives Secretariat found 175 health co-operatives across the country in 2010.[13] The data provide information on the nature of services offered by these co-operatives as well as the geographic location in which they are situated. Information on the type of co-operative (for example, consumer-driven versus worker-owned) was not available through this source and instead was located through provincial government departments and research reports.

These data reveal several trends. One is that health co-operatives have not proliferated the way Rands and other clinic organizers had hoped. Even if one adds community health centres to this mix (as discussed by Kagis and Saunders in this volume), the model of care being delivered through private practice is still the predominant model of care delivery in Canada. Related to this point is that the development of health co-operatives is regional, with 39 out of 58 clinics located in Quebec. The remaining clinics are evenly distributed across all other provinces except Newfoundland and Labrador. The development of new health co-operatives is also quite recent, with 30 incorporated in Quebec between 2006 and 2009.[14]

A second trend is that consumer-oriented health co-operatives have expanded to different health services beyond primary care. While the survey indicates that there are 58 health clinics across the country, there is also nearly the same number of co-operatives offering home care services. Most of these organizations are offering supportive services to the elderly and disabled, including assistance with housekeeping and meal preparation. Similar to health clinics, these home support co-operatives are located primarily in Quebec,[15] and developed as a result of a government initiative introduced in 1997 to both create jobs and address unmet demand for supportive services.[16]

Beyond home support services, co-operatives have also been organized by and for individuals with mental health disabilities. These organizations typically offer members peer support in a non-clinical environment; the purpose of these organizations is to provide non-judgmental and accepting spaces where individuals facing shared challenges can meet. These organizations may also deliver employment training and operate social enterprises as pathways to better mental health. The boards of directors of these co-operatives consist either entirely or predominantly of consumers/survivors of the mental health system.[17]

A third and important trend that has developed since the emergence of the community clinic movement is a new governance model within health co-operatives. This model challenges consumer sponsorship as advocated by Rands and other organizers of the co-operative clinics in Saskatchewan since it places consumers directly alongside other stakeholders at the board table. These organizations are called "multi-stakeholder" or "solidarity" co-operatives, and they are notably present among health clinics[18] and home support co-operatives[19] in Quebec. In multi-stakeholder co-operatives, more than one interest group is involved in governing the organization. Beyond consumers, stakeholder groups may include health care providers, such as doctors or front line workers, and supporting members, who are individuals or representatives from groups that champion the work of the co-operative.[20] Within these multi-stakeholder organizations, an overarching organizational purpose is shared, and each stakeholder group brings its experiences and perspectives to the table in order to accomplish common goals.

This trend toward "multi-stakeholderism" is different from the co-operative model of health care delivery as developed in Saskatchewan. Although staff have the opportunity to participate in the governance of the community clinics, it is an optional component rather than a structural aspect of these organizations. This means that worker participation may ebb and flow over time[21]; it may also be issue-based, where staff become involved when they are motivated or inspired by particular challenges they would like to see addressed through the board of directors.[22] In solidarity co-operatives, the involvement of more than one stakeholder group in governance is a permanent, structural feature.

An additional trend among co-operative clinics offering primary care is that the form of doctor remuneration so fiercely challenged by Rands is typically no longer part of the debate regarding the delivery of services. In Quebec, where survey data indicate the development of co-operative clinics has been the most robust, doctors involved in these organizations continue working on a fee-for-service basis. The main goal of these co-operatives is not to fundamentally reshape how health care is delivered, but to attract and retain health care providers to their communities by owning buildings and renting space to doctors.[23]

But although it may appear as though the role of these co-operatives is simply to act as landlords, there is in fact some overlap with the community clinic model in Saskatchewan in terms of approach to service delivery. In fact, these organizations typically endeavor to create spaces not just for physicians, but for allied professionals, such as physiotherapists and nutritionists.[24] Further, some of these organizations are involved in addressing the social determinants of health by working on projects such as community gardens and housing development. As such, like the Saskatchewan clinics, they may offer a range of primary care services to consumers and also be preventative in their approach to health.

Finally, it is important to note that although these new co-operatives are not organizing against a medical association or the private practice model of care delivery, they are working to counter interests of other kinds. For one, co-operative developers and advocates in Quebec argue that large corporations entice doctors away from smaller communities by offering them office space in buildings where these companies own and operate drug stores, with the hope that patients fill their prescriptions at the adjoining pharmacies. These buildings are located in communities where the population is large enough to offer an adequate market share to these corporations, leaving smaller communities underserviced by doctors.[25] Health co-operatives, as a result, are serving as a community-based response to this phenomenon. A second phenomenon to which organizers of health co-operatives are reacting is outmigration: these facilities are seen as providing necessary services that will help curb the potential exodus of younger people and the elderly to larger communities.[26]

Opportunities and Challenges

Despite the fact that the co-operative model of health care delivery has not grown in the way that early organizers had hoped, there are individuals and organizations across the country which are as committed as the Saskatchewan pioneers regarding the development of health co-operatives that feature either consumer control or, in the case of multi-stakeholder co-operatives, consumer involvement. These advocates and co-operative developers face a number of opportunities and challenges in advancing their work.

One such challenge is that co-operatives may be constrained by government policy regarding how the funding provided to them should be spent, thereby limiting the true ability for consumers to make substantive decisions regarding the nature of the services offered to them. Those involved in the early days of the community clinic movement in Saskatchewan understood this limitation, and successfully argued that global budgets were required so that individual co-operatives could plan programs and services that met the needs of their members.[27] Newer co-operatives operating in other jurisdictions have not always been able to make this case: in Quebec, for example, government funding is only available to pay for certain specific services offered by home support co-operatives; any potential new services identified by consumers fall beyond the parameters of the program and are not eligible for financial support.[28]

Establishing partnerships with provincial and territorial governments for the delivery of a wider range of health care services is a second challenge faced by health co-operatives. Such services include operating laboratories, diagnostic facilities, long-term care homes and surgical clinics. Many jurisdictions across Canada are privatizing service delivery through contracts with the for-profit sector[29]; governments argue that this contracting cuts back on the higher cost of public delivery and reduces the length of time patients must wait for care.[30] Here the challenge is that the co-operative model is not considered an alternative service delivery vehicle,[31] even though community clinics in Saskatchewan, for example, have had successful track records operating laboratories, pharmacies and performing minor surgeries.

While co-operative developers and associations may contend that the problem is lack of awareness regarding the co-operative form,[32] the true challenge is arguably a lack of commitment on the part of policy makers to a system of shared governance with social economy organizations.[33] One example of such a commitment occurred with the development of the home support co-operatives in Quebec in the 1990s: before that point, these social economy organizations were not active in the home support sector in that province. Still, the government was committed to delivery through certain organizational types and provided funding so that new co-operatives (as well as non-profits) could become established. For-profit businesses, on the other hand, were excluded from this collaboration. Moreover, the provincial government also committed to amending the co-operative legislation at that time in response to the community sector's interest in the development of multi-stakeholder co-operatives for the delivery of home support—as well as other—services.[34]

A third challenge that faces the new development of co-operative health care organizations that feature consumer involvement in governance is that the sector must be able to make a case regarding the adoption of its specific organizational form versus the development of community-based health care organizations which are also non-profit in nature. For example, although co-operative clinics were developed in Saskatchewan in the 1960s, the province of Ontario introduced community health centres a decade later; these centres overlap almost completely with community clinics in their objectives and approach to care.[35] But while this health centre model features citizen boards, directors do not have to be users of health centre services. Rather, potential directors are recruited with specific skill sets, as well as to reflect the socio-demographic and cultural composition of the communities in which they are located.[36]

Co-operatives are in a position to articulate a difference, however, in that a growing body of evidence supports direct user involvement in the governance of health care services. Herein lies a first opportunity for the sector. In the case of consumer-controlled mental health organizations, for example, research has found that individuals involved in such associations experience less anxiety and depression, decreased hospital stays, fewer doctors' visits, and less use of outpatient and crisis services. Individuals with mental health disabilities also report that they derive greater benefits from this model compared to both hospital care and programming delivered from other community-based providers that are not user-driven. Further, the fact that decision-making is controlled by users of these mental health services has been found to be an integral component to the success of these organizations.[37] In the home support sector, research has also shown that having consumers on the board of directors is associated with the quality of care provided.[38]

Despite this evidence linking user involvement in governance to positive outcomes, it is important to note that this does introduce a tension for health co-operatives. Specifically, differentiating the organizational form from other community-based health centres may undermine the advocacy work done by promoters of a model of primary care delivery that features salaried providers offering interdisciplinary services through non-profit organizations of different types (that is, non-profit or co-operative). Divisions of this kind have been argued to make partnerships with government more difficult, as policy makers may be unsure as to which organizations, exactly, should be convened in consultations and dialogue. Such is the case in Quebec as the system of shared governance between the government and the social economy sector currently weakens: observers have pointed to the divisions between the provincial co-operative sector and the *Chantier de l'économie sociale*, an umbrella association representing social economy organizations in Quebec, as one cause.[39]

Another opportunity for consumer-governed co-operative health care is that the organizational form has a track record of innovating in the realm of service delivery. This is an important characteristic of co-operatives as policy makers search for ways to make the health care system more responsive to changing demographics and emerging health care needs. Small scale innovations allow for new programs and services to be tested and potentially funded or scaled up by government if successful; two noted historical examples developed by the Saskatchewan co-operatives include podiatry services and a drug plan.[40] Current examples include the Saskatoon Community Clinic taking on a leadership role in providing services to an escalating number of individuals in the city infected with HIV/AIDS: their work has involved developing in-house processes and expertise on how to manage and treat infected patients[41] as well as moving their inner city clinic into an expanded facility. The provincial government has since responded by providing funding for a new doctor and to help cover new infrastructure costs incurred by the clinic.[42] As a second example, a web site developed by the co-operative sector in Nova Scotia allows consumers to access health information, establish personal health records, and communicate electronically with participating doctors' offices. This initiative represents the sector's efforts to make the health care system in that province both more consumer-centred and web-focused.[43]

Addressing the profit orientation of private clinics was a major focus for Rands and other clinic organizers; here the concern was whether an appropriate focus would be placed on addressing the health needs of patients. Salaried doctors were seen as the solution to this issue, and this type of remuneration remains an important feature of Saskatchewan community clinics. However, a related opportunity now exists for consumer-governed co-operatives regarding health care financing: escalating health care costs combined with an overall interest in transparency and accountability among policy makers[44] means that the openness afforded by the co-operative form is important, at least compared to corporations receiving public funding to deliver services. Co-operatives must, by law, provide users of their services with access to annual reports and financial statements.[45] Moreover, members' meetings provide consumers with the opportunity to ask specific questions related to these documents, including queries related to wages and benefits provided to staff and management, the organization's operating costs, and the generation and use of any surplus revenue. Research regarding potential efficiencies related to the co-operative form is a related opportunity, but should not be conflated with simple transparency regarding how public funding is spent by private health care providers. Co-operatives have an important opportunity to set a standard of openness for the health care sector and to take a leadership role in the debate regarding the use of public funding.

Stan Rands served as the executive director of a provincial association of community clinics that worked to recruit doctors and to advocate to Saskatchewan policy makers; this association evolved into a provincial federation and continues to serve as a venue through which existing clinics can communicate with the provincial government, discuss shared challenges and educate individuals and organizations about their model of health care delivery. In the summer of 2011, a national federation was founded to bridge health co-operatives of different kinds, including those offering primary care, home care, and services and supports for mental health consumers/survivors. This new federation presents an additional opportunity for the sector, as it allows members to learn about different kinds of health co-operatives and the enabling conditions for their development, and provides members with the opportunity to exchange expertise and lessons learned.[46]

Stan Rands refers to the rise of community clinics in Saskatchewan in the 1960s as a movement. As he explained in chapter one, the ability to organize quickly in the health care sector in response to the doctors' strike was a result both of mutual health plans that had predated the clinics, as well as the experience that organizers had developed while establishing co-operative infrastructure and consumer control in other sectors of the economy, including banking and retail stores. An additional element that facilitated this movement was the contribution of financial resources from other co-operative sectors; for example, it is noteworthy that when the provincial association of community clinics closed its doors, its significant debt was paid by two large co-operative businesses unrelated to the health care sector: the Saskatchewan Wheat Pool, a producer co-operative, and Federated Co-operatives Limited, a second tier organization which supplies retail co-operatives in the prairies.[47] This movement dimension is enshrined in two of the principles which define co-operative organizations: education about the model, and co-operation among co-operatives.[48]

It is this movement dimension that remains a final, and important, opportunity for health co-operatives today. It allows for information, expertise and resources to be shared in order to strengthen and further develop health care delivery through this organizational form. Health care providers incorporated as proprietary businesses do not constitute a movement; non-profit associations offering health care services are also not linked to other non-profit organizations as a matter of principle or to further the expansion of the non-profit sector.

Currently, the movement dimension of co-operatives can be seen at the local level when credit unions offer financing and technical assistance to help with the start-up of health co-operatives.[49] It can also be seen at the provincial and national levels through second and third-tier co-operative associations such as the Saskatchewan Co-operative Association and the Canadian Co-operative Association. These associations bring together co-operatives from different sectors, such as health, housing, agriculture, retail and social care services, and provide leadership training, facilitate information sharing, and promote public policies that favour co-operative development. Finally, this movement dimension can be found at the global level through the International Co-operative Alliance (ICA), the largest non-governmental organization in the world. The ICA unites health co-operatives worldwide with other co-operative sectors and, like its national and provincial counterparts, also provides training and information sharing.

It is noteworthy that the year 2012 not only represents the 50th anniversary of medicare and the Saskatchewan community clinics, but also the International Year of Co-operatives.[50] This declaration, made by the United Nations, recognizes the role that co-operatives of all kinds play in the economic and social development of communities around the globe, and it may serve as a catalyst for expanded co-operative development in the health sector.

Notes

1. For example, see the Co-operative Health Centre Prince Albert, 48th Annual Meeting Report, 2010: 8; Community Health Services Association (Saskatoon) Limited, "Advocacy," retrieved October 6, 2011, from http://www.saskatooncommunityclinic.ca/.

2. See Brett Fairbairn, "The Co-operative Tradition in Canada," in John Restakis and Evert A. Lindquist (eds.), *The Co-op Alternative: Civil Society and the Future of Public Services* (Toronto: The Institute of Public Administration in Canada, 2001), 41–42; Douglas E. Angus and Pran Manga, *Co-op/Consumer Sponsored Health Care Delivery Effectiveness* (Ottawa: Canadian Co-operative Association, 1990).

3. See also Samuel Wolfe, "Saskatchewan Community Clinics," *Canadian Medical Association Journal* 91 (1964): 225–29; Dennis Gruending, *The First Ten Years* (Saskatoon: Saskatoon Community Clinic, 1974).

4. International Co-operative Alliance, "Statement on the Co-operative Identity," retrieved October 6, 2011, from http://www.ica.coop/.

5. Government of Canada, *Canada Cooperatives Act 1998*, c. 7, s. 1, retrieved October 6, 2011, from http://laws-lois.justice.gc.ca.

6. For Saskatchewan, see Government of Saskatchewan, *The Co-operative's Act 1998*, c. 37.3, s. 3, retrieved October 6, 2011, from http://nslegislature.ca/.

7. For example, see Community Health Services Association (Regina) Limited, *Bylaws of Community Health Services Association (Regina) Limited*, 2001; Community Health Services Association (Saskatoon), *Bylaws of Community Health Services Association (Saskatoon) Limited* (n.d.).

8. Legislation pertaining to health services co-operatives in Saskatchewan in fact allows staff to hold up to one third of total board seats if they in fact choose to become actively involved in decision-making at this level (Government of Saskatchewan, *The Co-operative's Act 1998*, c. 37.3, s. 268, retrieved October 6, 2011, from http://nslegislature.ca/.) However, the extent to which staff members participate varies. The Prince Albert clinic, for example, currently has one staff member on the board of directors (personal communication, Bonnie Peneff with author, October 5, 2011), as does the Regina Community Clinic (personal communication, Lesley Crossman with author, October 12, 2011). The Saskatoon and Wynyard clinics currently have no staff on their boards (personal communication, Coreen Usselman with author, October 5, 2011 and Shirley Yewsuk with author, October 12, 2011). Further, regardless of whether staff is involved in governance, consumers still hold a majority voice at the board table.

9. See the Community Health Services Association (Saskatoon) Limited, *Saskatoon Community Clinic Year in Review*, 2010–2011; Co-operative Health Centre Prince Albert, 48th *Annual Meeting Report*, 2010; Community Health Services Association (Regina) Limited, *Annual Report*, 2010–2011.

10. Community Health Services Association (Saskatoon) Limited, "Resolutions–CHSA Annual Meeting–June 21, 2011," retrieved October 6, 2011, from http://www.saskatooncommunityclinic.ca/.

11. The different relationships boards of directors may have with management are summarized by Chris Cornforth, "The Governance of Cooperatives and Mutual Associations: A Paradox Perspective," *Annals of Public and Cooperative Economics* 75, no. 1 (2004): 11–32.

12. For example, Christian Jetté and Benoît Lévesque, "Les rapports de consommation et la participation des usagers," in Yves Vaillancourt, François Aubry and Christian Jetté (eds.), *L'économie sociale dans les services à domicile* (Quebec: Presses de l'Université du Québec, 2003), 151–200 and Moira Lees and Reimer Volkers, "General Trends, Findings and Recommendations," *Review of International Co-operation,* 89, no. 4 (1996): 37–49.

13. Data were received by the author through e-mail from Marylène Gagné, Senior Data Analyst, Rural and Co-operatives Secretariat, February 2011.

14. Marie-Joëlle Brassard, Patrice Leblanc and Olivier Ėtienne, *Les coopératives de santé au Québec: Du consommateur à l'acteur !* (Rimouski: Cahiers de l'ARUC – Développement territorial et coopération, Série «Recherche» numéro 5, 2009), 16.

15. Régie de l'assurance maladie Québec, "Liste des entreprises d'économie sociale en aide domestique (EESAD)," retrieved October 11, 2011, from http://www.ramq.gouv.qc.ca/.

16. In 1996, representatives from government, women's organizations, labour unions and the community sector determined that non-profit and co-operative organizations could create jobs in underdeveloped but growing markets such as home support. These services were not being offered by other health care providers in the province. Yves Vaillancourt and Christian Jetté (with the assistance of Philippe Leclerc), *Les arrangements institutionnels entre l'État québécois et les entreprises d'économie sociale en aide domestique : Une analyse sociopolitique de l'économie sociale dans les services de soutien à domicile* (Montréal: Les éditions vie économique, 2009): 31–37.

17. See Julia Bidonde and Catherine Leviten-Reid, *A Place to Learn, Work and Heal: An Evaluation of Crocus Co-operative* (Saskatoon: Community University Institute for Social Research, University of Saskatchewan, 2011), 1–2.

18. Brassard, Leblanc and Ėtienne, *Les coopératives de santé au Québec*, 29–30.

19. Régie de l'assurance maladie Québec, Liste des entreprises d'économie sociale en aide domestique (EESAD)," retrieved October 11, 2011, from http://www.ramq.gouv.qc.ca/.

20. Éditeur officiel du Québec, *Loi sur les Coopératives* 2011, c. 7, s. 226.1, retrieved October 14, 2011, from http://www2.publicationsduQuébec.gouv.qc.ca/.

21. Interview, Patrick Lapointe with author, November 25, 2009.

22. Personal communication, Lesley Crossman with author, October 12, 2011.

23. Brassard, Leblanc and Ėtienne, *Les coopératives de santé au Québec*, 14 and 17. In Quebec, Local Community Service Centres (or CLSs) were established in the early 1970s. They offer inter-professional primary care services through salaried physicians. Claude Sicotte, Danielle D'Amour and Marie-Pierre Moreault, "Interdisciplinary Collaboration Within Québec Community Health Care Centres," *Social Science & Medicine* 55, no. 6 (2002): 991–1003.

24. Brassard, Leblanc and Ėtienne, *Les coopératives de santé au Québec*, 29.

25. Jean Pierre Girard, *Implementation of a Health Services Co-operative: Factors for Success and Failure* (Ottawa: Co-operatives Secretariat, 2005), 1.

26. Brassard, Leblanc and Ėtienne, *Les coopératives de santé au Québec*, 19.

27. Gruending, *The First Ten Years*, 21–22.

28. Régie de l'assurance maladie Québec, "Quels sont les services d'aide domestique visés?," retrieved October 11, 2011, from http://www.ramq.gouv.qc.ca/.

29. British Columbia Medical Association, Public-private Partnerships (P3s) in Health Care, 2010: 1–2.

30. For example, Province of Saskatchewan, *Sooner, Safer, Smarter: A Plan to Transform the Surgical Patient Experience* (The Author, 2010): 11.

31. See John Restakis and Evert A. Lindquist, "Introduction: Government Restructuring and

the Co-operative Alternative," in John Restakis and Evert A. Lindquist (eds.), *The Co-op Alternative: Civil Society and the Future of Public Services* (Toronto: The Institute of Public Administration in Canada, 2001), 10.

32. See John Anderson, "Health co-ops and the future of Medicare," *Making Waves* 18, no. 3 (2007): 40–42.

33. The term "shared governance" is based on Susan Phillips, *The Intersection of Governance and Citizenship in Canada: Not Quite the Third Way* (Montréal: Institute for Research on Public Policy, 2006).

34. Yves Vaillancourt and Christian Jetté (with the assistance of Philippe Leclerc). *Les arrangements institutionnels*, 36.

35. Ministry of Health and Long Term Care Ontario, *Community Health Centre Policy and Procedures Manual* (The Author, 2001): 5–6.

36. Ibid., 10. The province of Quebec also introduced similar organizations in the 1970s, called Local Community Service Centres (or CLSCs), a move which supplanted the work of a small number of grassroots clinics that had emerged in the province in the 1960s. Frédéric Leseman, *Services and Circuses: Community and the Welfare State* (Montreal: Black Rose Books, 1984), 239–41. The CLSCs operated as stand-alone non-profit organizations until the provincial government restructured health care services in 2003–04. The CLSCs now fall under the purview of the *centres de santé et de services sociaux* (CSSS) along with hospitals and long-term care facilities. Santé et Services sociaux Québec, "Centres de santé et de services sociaux," retrieved October 12, 2011 from http://www.msss.gouv.qc.ca/. CLSCs no longer have their own boards of directors; there is one board for each CSSS. Yves Vaillancourt and Christian Jetté (with the assistance of Philippe Leclerc), *Les arrangements institutionnels*, 49.

37. See Carol Mowbray and Cheribeth Tan, "Consumer-operated Drop-in Centers: Evaluation of Operations and Impact," *The Journal of Mental Health Administration* 20, no. 1 (1993): 8–19; Geoff Nelson, Joanna Ochocka, Rich Janzen, John Trainor, Paula Goering, and Jonathan Lomotey, "A Longitudinal Study of Mental Health Consumer/Survivor Initiatives: Part V – Outcomes at 3-year Follow-up," Journal of Community Psychology 35, no. 5 (2007): 655–65; Joanna Ochocka, Geoff Nelson, Rich Janzen, and John Trainor, "A Longitudinal Study of Mental Health Consumer/Survivor Initiatives: Part 3–A Qualitative Study of Impacts of Participation on New Members," *Journal of Community Psychology* 34, no.3 (2006): 273–83.

38. Catherine Leviten-Reid and Ann Hoyt, "Community-based Home Support Agencies: Comparing the Quality of Care of Cooperative and Non-profit Agencies," *Canadian Journal on Aging* 28, no. 2 (2009): 107–20.

39. Yves Vaillancourt and Christian Jetté (with the assistance of Philippe Leclerc), *Les arrangements institutionnels*, 112.

40. Brett Fairbairn, "The Co-operative Tradition in Canada," in John Restakis and Evert A. Lindquist (eds.), *The Co-op Alternative: Civil Society and the Future of Public Services* (Toronto: The Institute of Public Administration in Canada, 2001), 41.

41. Interview, Cheryl Hand with author, January 13, 2010.

42. Laurie Stone, "Westside Clinic Expands Care for HIV/AIDS Patients," *Focus* 46, no. 3 (2010): 3.

43. Nova Scotia Co-operative Council, "HealthConnex Health Care Initative," retrieved October 14, 2011, from http://www.nsco-opcouncil.ca/.

44. For example, see Government of Canada, *Federal Accountability Action Plan: Turning a New Leaf* (Ottawa: Author, 2006).

45. Government of Canada, *Canada Cooperatives Act 1998*, c. 247, s. 1, retrieved October 6, 2011, from http://laws-lois.justice.gc.ca.

46. Personal communication, Mark Goldblatt with author, March 30 and August 8, 2011.

47. Gruending, *The First Ten Years*, 10.

48. International Co-operative Alliance, "Statement on the Co-operative Identity," retrieved October 6, 2011, from http://www.ica.coop/.

49. M-J. Brassard, P. Leblanc and O. Ėtienne, "Les coopératives de santé au Québec," 17 and 21.

50. United Nations General Assembly A/Res/64/136, 2010, "Cooperatives in Social Development." Retrieved October 12, 2010, from http://www.un.org/.

Index

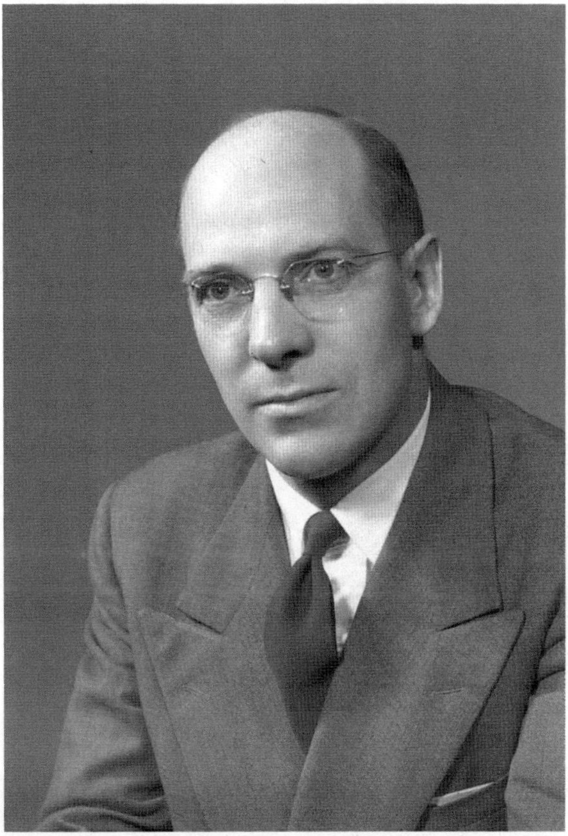

A Rhodes scholar, Stan Rands worked as a senior civil servant in the Psychiatric Services Branch of the Department of Public Health in Saskatchewan for over a decade before becoming the first executive director of the Community Health Service (Sask) Association months after the Doctors' Strike of 1962. For the next decade, he recruited new doctors who were sympathetic to the ideals of the community clinics and he struggled in favour of a physician payment system that would encourage better care for patients. In his later years, he was a university professor and community clinic board member as well as social justice activist. Stan Rands died in 1985.

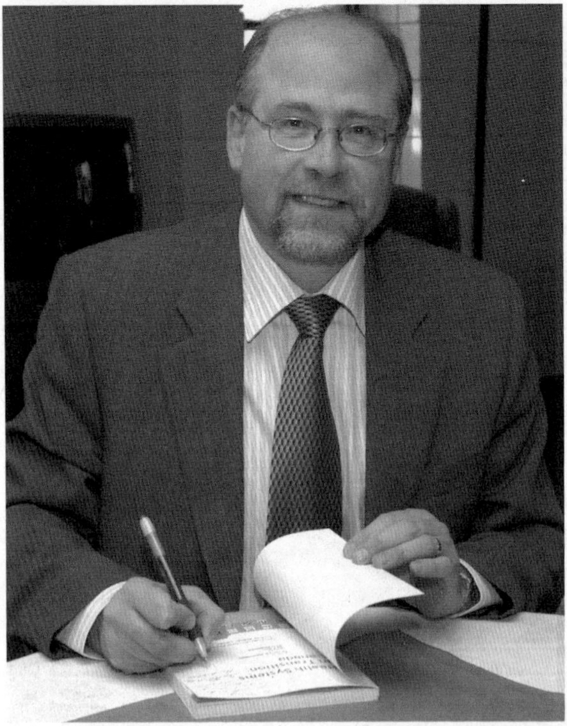

Gregory P. Marchildon is a Canada Research Chair and Professor in the Johnson-Shoyama Graduate School of Public Policy and is the author of a number of books on Canadian history and public policy. After receiving his PhD from the London School of Economics, Marchildon taught for five years at Johns Hopkins University. He returned to Saskatchewan in 1994 to become a deputy minister in the provincial government and was cabinet secretary and deputy minister to the premier from 1996 until 2000. From 2001 until 2002, he served as the executive director of the Royal Commission on the Future of Health Care in Canada led by Roy Romanow.

Catherine Leviten-Reid is an Assistant Professor in the Shannon School of Business, Cape Breton University, where she teaches in the MBA in Community Economic Development program. She does research on community enterprises that deliver health and social care. Catherine has a PhD in Human Ecology from the University of Wisconsin-Madison. She was a postdoctoral fellow at the Centre for the Study of Co-operatives, University of Saskatchewan, from 2008 to 2009, and served as a director of the Saskatoon Community Clinic from 2008 to 2010.

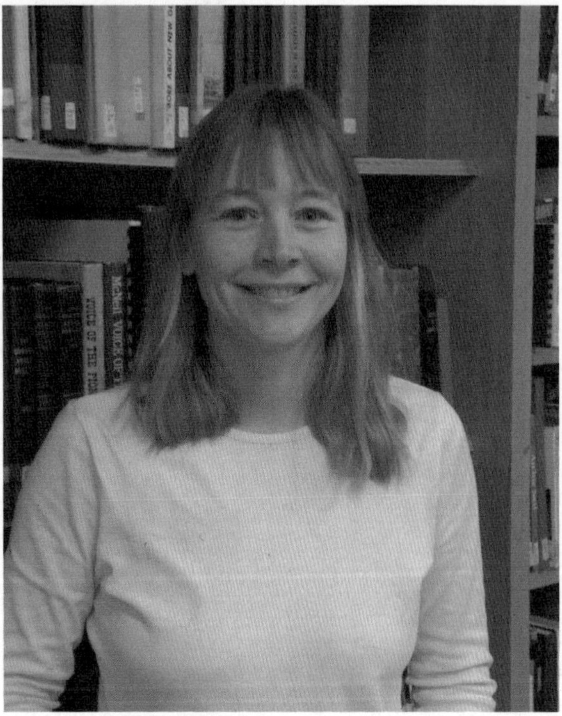